FIBROMYALGIA

THE NEW INTEGRATIVE APPROACH

How to Combine the Best of Traditional and Alternative Therapies

MILTON HAMMERLY, M.D.

Produced by The Philip Lief Group, Inc.

Adams Media Corporation

Holbrook, Massachusetts

For Joanie and Matthew,
my love for you is beyond measure.

Published by
Adams Media Corporation
260 Center Street, Holbrook, MA 02343 U.S.A.
www.adamsmedia.com

ISBN: 1-58062-464-2

Printed in Canada.

J I H G F E D C B A

Library of Congress Cataloging-in-Publication Data
Hammerly, Milton.
Fibromyalgia : the new integrative approach : how to combine the best of
traditional and alternative therapies / Milton Hammerly.
p.   cm.
ISBN 1-58062-464-2
1. Fibromyalgia. 2. Fibromyalgia--Alternative treatment. I. Title.
RC927.3.H35   2000
616.7'4--dc21   00-038126
CIP

Many of the designations used by manufacturers and sellers to distinguish
their products are claimed as trademarks. Where those designations
appear in this book and Adams Media was aware of a trademark claim,
the designations have been printed in initial capital letters.

This publication is designed to provide accurate and authoritative
information with regard to the subject matter covered. It is sold with
the understanding that the publisher is not engaged in rendering
professional medical advice. If assistance is required, the services of a
competent professional person should be sought.

This book is available at quantity discounts for bulk
purchases. For information, call 1-800-872-5627.

Acknowledgments

This book would not have been possible without an able team of writers and researchers that included Carol Sorgen, Carol Coughlin, R.D., Rebecca Valentine, and Cindy Spitzer, and the patience and skill of Rhonda Heisler and Lynne Kirk of The Philip Lief Group, who wove together the many threads into a cohesive whole. Thanks also to the superb guiding hand of Cheryl Kimball, my editor at Adams Media Corporation.

Joanie, my wife and editor-in-residence, listened patiently and helped me sort through the innumerable ideas for this series.

I am deeply indebted to the many acupuncturists, chiropractors, herbalists, massage therapists, naturopaths, nutritionists, reflexologists, and other practitioners with whom I have been privileged to work over the years. These talented, dedicated health care providers have given me the opportunity to see medicine and the healing arts through different (nonsurgical and nonpharmaceutical) eyes.

I am equally grateful to my fellow physicians and hospital administrators who have supported me, even when my career strayed beyond the conines of medical textbooks and double-blind–placebo-controlled research. Your goodwill has kept me going many times when I have been tempted to quit.

For all the patients who have challenged me, stretched my skills, and taught me more than medical school about the art of medicine, I am both appreciative and humbled.

Finally, for circumstances totally beyond my control, for doors closing and doors opening, and for the faith to pass through those doors, I am eternally grateful.

Contents

Introduction

NOT YOUR STANDARD BOOK ON FIBROMYALGIA

If you've picked up this book among all the other books on fibromyalgia, you probably already have a healthy curiosity about what unconventional medicine has to offer.

In that respect you're part of a general population trend. A recent landmark issue of the *Journal of the American Medical Association (JAMA)* reported that over 40 percent of Americans had broadened their health care menu to include such out-of-the-mainstream specialties as stress-reduction techniques, massage, herbal medicine, acupuncture, and homeopathy. In the past decade, visits to nonmedical healers jumped 50 percent. In fact, Americans are spending a whopping $27 billion a year on complementary and alternative treatments, vitamins, herbs, and books—most of that out of their own pockets, since much of what's classified as "complementary" or "alternative" medicine (often abbreviated as CAM) is not covered by health insurance.

Just what's driving the move to a greater use of unconventional therapies? A number of factors come into play:

- Broader access to more and (sometimes) better health care information, thanks to an explosion of media attention and now, of course, the Internet.

- An ever-increasing interest in disease prevention, wellness strategies, and the quest for optimal health—exactly those areas where complementary medicine can deliver the greatest benefits.

- An increase in the number of people with chronic health problems—such as fibromyalgia, allergies, asthma, chronic fatigue syndrome, diabetes, and various autoimmune disorders—and their inability to find adequate or lasting relief from symptoms through conventional medical treatment.

- A search for more effective pain control techniques, minus the side effects that frequently accompany prescription medications.

- An increasing dissatisfaction with the hurried, impersonal approach that characterizes much of health care delivery today. Under managed care, a visit to your doctor's office might involve just 10 minutes with your primary-care physician, barely enough time to do anything more than diagnose and treat your immediate symptoms. In contrast, your appointment with a complementary practitioner might last 60 to 90 minutes and take a comprehensive "whole patient" approach.

- The CAM mindset that makes a patient an empowered and active partner in his or her own health care.

Historically, Western medicine and complementary/alternative medicine have had little to do with each other, except to throw stones at each other on a fairly regular basis. Guess who's been caught in the middle of this futile feud? The patients! Although more and more people are turning to complementary and alternative practitioners for at least some of their health care needs, more than 60 percent of the time they're not telling their physicians about it. Given the potential for unrecognized interactions and contraindications, not to mention the likely therapeutic benefits, it's certainly in everyone's best interest to promote collaboration and a sharing of information between CAM practitioners and conventional physicians. Combining the best of CAM with the best of Western medicine allows for better individualization of therapy, fewer side effects, and better outcomes.

DOESN'T WESTERN MEDICINE HAVE THE CURE FOR FIBROMYALGIA?

Are all fibromyalgia patients alike? Does everyone experience fibromyalgia in the same way? Should the treatment of fibromyalgia be the same for all patients? If you're reading this book, you know intuitively that the answers to these questions are NO! NO! and NO! Unfortunately for many years the medical community has been answering these questions YES! YES! and YES!

Much of the medical community is still struggling over the recognition of fibromyalgia as a legitimate diagnosis, let alone seeing the need for individualized treatment strategies. For the most part, the medical community offers fibromyalgia patients symptom treatment without correcting the underlying causes, since the causes of fibromyalgia are not well understood. Treating symptoms is not only less effective than dealing with underlying causes, it is often associated with increased discomfort from the side effects of treatment.

Given our poor understanding of fibromyalgia and the marginal success of conventional medical treatments in most cases, you would think physicians would be open to patients trying complementary and alternative approaches, since many times such interventions are more effective and better tolerated. Unfortunately, many physicians are not familiar with all that CAM has to offer. They simply tell patients there is "nothing else to do" and that trying CAM interventions would be "a waste of time and money." Not only is this advice uninformed, it is detrimental to patients whose lives have been impacted emotionally, financially, physically, socially, and spiritually by fibromyalgia. If physicians are unable to provide the solutions patients need, they should learn to actively collaborate with other disciplines that may have the needed answers, or at least not impede patients from seeking help elsewhere.

The fact that Western medicine does not have a cure for fibromyalgia does not constitute a failure. Where Western medicine fails is in not collaborating with other disciplines or recognizing that there are answers to be found elsewhere. The theories, teachings, and biases of Western medicine are often treated as if they were more important than finding solutions for suffering patients. This "med-centric" approach is somewhat akin to the pre-Copernican notion of the universe. Insisting that the sun revolves around the earth, instead of vice versa, is not too different from thinking that Western medicine is at the center of the health care universe and everything else revolves around it. If the goal of medicine is to serve rather than to be served, then the health of patients should be at the center of the health care universe.

With our attention diverted by all the cataclysmic changes occurring in health care (technological advancements, skyrocketing costs, government and insurance rules, and so on), the welfare of patients is too often pushed aside. The misplaced focus on "tech-centric," "cost-centric," "rule-centric" medicine leads to an increasingly unbalanced, dysfunctional, and sick health care system. There is only one cure for these ailments of focus. **The patient is the cure.**

INTEGRATIVE MEDICINE—
BRIDGING THE GAPS THROUGH
PATIENT-CENTERED CARE

This book is addressed to patients with fibromyalgia who are looking for answers that the medical community has not yet been willing or able to provide. Some of these answers are found in nutrition therapies, and many belong to the world of complementary and alternative medicine. The philosophy of *integrative medicine*—which recognizes the role of body, mind, and spirit in health; favors individualized, patient-centered care; and encourages the rational and judicious combination of conventional Western medicine *and* complementary and alternative medicine, based on evidence of both efficacy and safety—underlies all of the recommendations in this book. Armed with this information, patients with fibromyalgia can take a much more proactive role in their own health care.

Integrative medicine approaches patients with fibromyalgia using a more collaborative, more pragmatic "patient-centric" model, one that blends the best of what Western medicine has to offer with the best of the complementary therapies. This approach is grounded in the holistic understanding that people are unique. We all have different emotional, physical, social, and spiritual needs that affect or are affected by the state of our health. Integrative medicine puts the total well-being of the patient back in the center of the health care universe where it belongs.

Many patients with fibromyalgia have arrived at my office in desperation, having seen and tried every conventional medical approach available and experienced either marginal benefits or unacceptable side effects. They have been told repeatedly by their physicians that nothing else can be done and that they should "learn to live with it." My challenge has been to check for diagnostic and/or therapeutic "blind spots" that other doctors have been unwilling or unable to consider. This mere willingness to look for new explanations or try different approaches has proven to be therapeutic in and of itself. When patients understand that your approach centers around their total well-being and that your philosophy will not be an obstacle to their healing, the healing relationship can change dramatically.

WHY WESTERN MEDICINE DOESN'T HAVE ALL THE ANSWERS YOU NEED

As a conventionally trained, board-certified family practitioner, I know as well as any physician that the accomplishments of Western medicine in surgery, in infectious diseases, and in other health crises are nothing short of amazing. But as a doctor who specializes in treating people with chronic disorders, and one who often collaborates with complementary and alternative practitioners, I also know that conventional medicine does not have all the answers.

One problem is that conventionally trained doctors generally dismiss as "unscientific," "quackery," "irrelevant," or "dangerous" any therapy that has not been proven effective in double-blind–placebo-controlled (DBPC) research. There are several problems inherent in this position, the most obvious being that a majority of Western medical interventions have not met this standard. In fact, most of the treatments conventional physicians currently recommend to their patients are based on a consensus of opinion within the medical community, rather than on sound research that has met the DBPC standard.

Should patients, as the conventional medical community suggests, ignore potentially valuable complementary and alternative therapies with centuries, if not millennia, of clinically demonstrated effectiveness just because they do not meet the methodological criteria of academicians? Or should doctors acknowledge what their patients are proving on a daily basis—that many of these interventions work? Isn't it time to look for other standards of proof?

In some cases, of course, there are excellent studies that meet the most stringent criteria and show consistent benefits from complementary interventions in well defined situations. Often, however, what's missing is a theory or mechanism that explains the outcomes in scientific terms that conventionally trained physicians understand.

Many complementary and alternative therapies are based on "alternate" healing systems—some of them energy-based—that are difficult to evaluate if you've been schooled in the Western biochemical model of medicine. Often such therapies are impossible to adequately "blind" so that neither the patient nor the researcher knows who is being treated with what as data is collected.

Traditional acupuncture is an example of one such therapy. There can be no true placebo in a study of acupuncture, because acupuncture needles introduced in "sham" points still have physiologic effects. Research that compares patients treated with needles in actual acupuncture points to those with needles in sham points is actually comparing the effect of doing something with the effect *doing something different*—not the effect of doing something versus the effect of *doing "nothing"* (a placebo). Furthermore, in traditional acupuncture, needle placement is based on a highly individualized assessment of the patient. A research design that calls for the practitioner to use the same set of acupoints in treating all patients runs counter to the philosophy and theory of traditional Chinese medicine. Therefore, such a study, by its own design, actually invalidates itself.

Electrostatic massage (a therapy using static electricity to correct charge imbalances in the body) and the "Meyer's cocktail" (an intravenous infusion of calcium, magnesium, vitamin C, and B vitamins) are two more therapies that can be quite beneficial for symptoms of fibromyalgia, but which are impossible to blind for research purposes. In the case of the Meyer's cocktail, you can taste the vitamins as they are being infused and you feel a warm sensation as your blood vessels dilate. There is no way that you wouldn't know whether or not you're getting the treatment. In the case of electrostatic massage, there is no mistaking the sensation of static electricity.

It's ludicrous to insist such therapies are not worthy of study or are clinically worthless because they don't fit the DBPC methodology. To say that the only real clinical effects of any therapy are those that remain after subtracting out the placebo (mind–body) effect, unfairly and irrationally slams the door shut on many useful interventions. If we were to use only those therapies compatible with DBPC testing, both Western medicine and CAM would have much less to offer patients and the amount of unnecessary human suffering would increase significantly. The intellectual orphaning of therapies not compatible with DBPC testing does an injustice to both science and humanity.

A second problem that creates barriers to most of complementary and alternative medicine is that conventional Western medicine assumes that all patients respond to treatment essentially the same way. We doctors are taught in medical school that basic physiology doesn't vary much from person to person. This assumption is reinforced by medical research that controls for variables and treats all patients identically. Such research validates only those therapies that show a statistically significant response in a uniform population. Individuality (nonuniformity) is lost in such statistics, as are the effects of those therapies that benefit subsets of nonuniform individuals who are part of a larger population.

However, what we've come to understand from the human genome project and from other avenues of research is that patients are not robots or genetically identical clones. There are dramatic genetic, enzymatic, biochemical, and environmental differences among people that dictate risk factors, how well a given patient will respond to a given intervention, and possible side effects. Complementary and alternative practitioners have long recognized this fact and make highly individualized assessment and treatment the cornerstone of care.

MODERN MEDICINE—ART OR SCIENCE, BOTH OR NEITHER?

Medicine is often described as both an art and a science. Science is the art of wrestling with what we don't know. Curiosity drives scientists to postulate a theory and then use their creativity to develop ways to test the theory to see whether it is right or wrong.

Many of the physicians who are the most vocal critics of complementary and alternative medicine call themselves "scientists" but do no research of their own. They quote liberally from other people's research and shun what is unfamiliar, saying it hasn't been studied adequately. Such doctors rarely exhibit the open-minded curiosity needed to wrestle with the unknown. This is not science, it is hiding behind science in lockstep conformity out of fear of peer rejection, professional ostracism, or litigation.

This is not to say that these same physicians fail to understand the importance of the mind–body connection. Not at all. They can even quote the research that explains how thoughts, emotions, and moods profoundly impact physiology and health. Yet they rarely incorporate this knowledge into everyday patient care.

In the first place, many physicians feel that to delve into this "touchy–feely" area lessens their stature as scientists. Secondly, the process of medical education is a brutal one for most doctors. It trains us to deal with cold, hard, objective facts and to deny our own needs and emotions, including the relevance of these needs and emotions to our general well-being.

It's not hard to understand how physicians, who've had their emotional sensitivity beaten out of them by conventional medical training, would have a difficult time acknowledging the mind-body connection in their own lives, much less in the lives of their patients. In this respect the art of medicine has been dealt a serious blow. There can be no art without acknowledging the heart. And if medicine is to be practiced as an art *and* a science, physicians need both open hearts and open minds.

WHAT YOU'LL LEARN HERE

This book takes an integrative approach to the management of fibromyalgia. In doing so it presents the best conventional approaches, nutritional approaches, and complementary and alternative approaches. I make no attempt to either avoid or create controversy. Where there is controversy relative to fibromyalgia, different perspectives are presented and common sense is applied in order to arrive at a balanced, collaborative approach that has your best interest in mind.

In no way do I wish to discount the role of conventional medicine in diagnosing and treating patients with fibromyalgia. After all, as a family practitioner, my own clinical practice falls squarely within this model. At the same time, my role as director of integrative medicine for Catholic Health Initiatives (a national hospital system with its headquarters in Denver), allows me to dialogue and collaborate on an ongoing basis with both physicians and CAM colleagues in Colorado and across the United States.

The opening chapters of this book cover fibromyalgia and related health issues from the conventional perspective, including some unconventional uses of conventional therapies. Then we present the case for sound nutrition and lifestyle strategies—both for optimal long-term health and to alleviate many of the most troubling symptoms of fibromyalgia. Several chapters are devoted to a discussion of the use of complementary therapies in fibromyalgia. Finally, we offer strategies for putting it all together in ways that make the most sense for you as an individual. I'll discuss my own "less-is-more" approach and provide some useful guidelines for coordinating care between your conventional physicians and your CAM practitioners.

WHY SHOULD YOU SEEK YET ANOTHER PERSPECTIVE ON FIBROMYALGIA?

That's a good question. No single person, therapy, or discipline has all of the answers to fibromyalgia. Fortunately, the perspective presented here is much more than my own. As a team of writers with expert knowledge of conventional medicine, complementary modalities, and nutrition, we've pulled together scientific theory and standard medical and nutritional practice with the real life experience of patients and the clinical know-how of many CAM practitioners.

As a physician who strives to listen carefully to my patients and learn from them, I've found that people with fibromyalgia are far better instructors on the realities of the disorder than are medical textbooks and journals. In that sense, the experience and wisdom of my patients—and in some cases, their complementary and alternative care providers—are also speaking to you through the pages of this book.

—MILTON HAMMERLY, M.D.
Denver, Colorado

1

Your Pain Has a Name—
Fibromyalgia:
The Inside Story

Maybe you hurt all over. Maybe you wake up every morning more exhausted than when you went to sleep. Maybe the muscle spasms, joint pain, headaches, and crushing fatigue have gotten so bad you can no longer raise your children, make love, hold a job, or lead a productive life. Or maybe you're just a little more achy and tired than you used to be . . . *and it isn't going away.*

Whether your life has become a living hell, or just moderately uncomfortable a bit longer than you expected, you may be among the six to 10 million Americans who suffer to varying degrees from a baffling variety of painful symptoms collectively referred to as *fibromyalgia.*

Only recently recognized by the conventional medical community as a "real" illness, fibromyalgia typically strikes adults in the prime of life, although more and more young people are also now being diagnosed. Female sufferers outnumber males at least three to one. Of course, women are more likely than men to seek health care and so are more likely to be identified. But, whether they know it or not, plenty of men suffer with it, too. In fact, by some estimates, only half of all adults with fibromyalgia have a name for their pain.

While not life-threatening, fibromyalgia can wreak havoc on your health and well-being, causing debilitating pain, depression, and a whole host of physical disturbances—from digestive problems to brain fog. To make matters worse, most mainstream doctors either completely ignore the problem, say it's all in your head, or mistake it for other illnesses. Patients "lucky" enough to get diagnosed correctly are often prescribed ineffective, sometimes dangerous drugs and other useless or inappropriate treatments.

Like many Americans, people with fibromyalgia are turning in increasing numbers to nontraditional health care—a collection of prevention strategies and interventions grouped under the heading complementary/alternative medicine (CAM). These practices include a wide variety of noninvasive, yet effective approaches, several of which are ideally suited for coping with chronic illnesses like fibromyalgia.

Even so, relying *entirely* on hit-or-miss CAM practices—perhaps the occasional massage, or a little herbal therapy—isn't particularly useful either. With so many alternative health modalities to pick from and so little research on what treatments work best for which illnesses, it's hard to find effective, long-term relief.

Fortunately this is changing. We are witnessing the birth of a new specialty which recognizes that individual uniqueness of mind, body, and spirit impacts health in powerful ways. This new specialty also recognizes the inadequacy of any one healing system to provide all the answers needed for optimal health. Using available scientific knowledge and a holistic understanding of the human condition allows us to weave together the best of both worlds—taking what works from conventional Western medicine and combining it with the most effective CAM practices. This emerging new specialty is called *integrative medicine*. Integrative medicine is by nature holistic, individualized, collaborative, and, above all, patient-centered.

As a physician trained in conventional medicine and highly experienced in complementary and alternative health practices, I have spent several years developing what I believe to be a rational, judicious approach to the diagnosis and treatment of fibromyalgia and other chronic illnesses. By focusing on each patient as a unique individual, taking a detailed history, identifying underlying associated disorders, and developing a treatment strategy that involves *both* conventional and complementary treatments, integrative medicine can do what neither Western medicine nor nontraditional practices can do on their own.

Living day in and day out with the chronic pain, crushing fatigue, and other debilitating symptoms of fibromyalgia can leave you feeling like a prisoner of your own life. With integrative medicine, you, your doctor, and your CAM practitioners work as a team, exploring multiple paths to greater comfort and freedom.

IT'S *NOT* ALL IN YOUR HEAD

The American College of Rheumatology and the National Institutes of Health estimate that six to 10 million Americans have fibromyalgia. But with so many people going undiagnosed, the actual number may be much higher.

Fibromyalgia strikes adults and children of every age, race, nationality, and socioeconomic group. Most people with fibromyalgia are diagnosed while in their twenties, thirties, and forties, but children as young as five have also been identified. Although about 85 to 90 percent of adults diagnosed with the condition are women, some clinicians believe fibromyalgia occurs just as frequently in men but goes unrecognized by many male patients and their physicians.

Often people with fibromyalgia live with the problem for many years while their symptoms first come and go, and then, eventually, come and stay. Some researchers say the average time between the onset of constant symptoms and receiving an *accurate* diagnosis is four or five years. During this time, many people with fibromyalgia bounce from one physician to another, searching for answers. Because so few doctors recognize fibromyalgia when they see it, and because the condition resembles, and even overlaps with, so many other health problems, fibromyalgia is often missed or misdiagnosed. When lab tests come back normal or inappropriate treatments fail, it's not uncommon to be told (or to be treated as if) "it's all in your head."

Well, it's *not* all in your head. In fact, it's all in your body—all *through* your body, potentially affecting many different systems, including your:

- Musculoskeletal system
- Digestive system
- Immune system
- Circulatory system
- Endocrine system
- Nervous system

To dismiss the far-reaching, multiple symptoms of fibromyalgia as being psychosomatic is not only insulting, it's potentially dangerous. A missed or incorrect diagnosis can lead to worsening symptoms and expose you to the unnecessary risks of improper treatments.

SYMPTOMS GALORE

Because fibromyalgia has no single, known cause it is not a "diagnosis" in the strictest sense of the word. The "gnosis" in diagnosis implies an understanding or knowledge of the causes involved. It may be that many different underlying conditions can cause the same cluster of symptoms we refer to as fibromyalgia. If this is the case, patients with fibromyalgia need to be treated as a heterogeneous group with similar symptoms, rather than a homogenous group that responds to a "one size fits all" approach. If fibromyalgia is considered a diagnosis that describes a homogenous group of patients, it may actually do these patients a disservice. Therefore, since the underlying causes can vary and are not well understood, it is best to think of "fibromyalgia" as a label used to describe a *syndrome*—that is, a group of signs and symptoms.

Fibromyalgia is characterized by two different types of pain. The first type is widespread, diffused, chronic muscle pain (often described as flu-like) that comes and goes or stays constant throughout the body. The second type involves specific "tender points" of pain. Press on a tender point and the person suffering from fibromyalgia experiences an intense, knuckle-whitening pain, but only in the spot where pressure is directly applied.

In addition to widespread pain and "tender point" pain, people with fibromyalgia may suffer from one or more additional symptoms—an often confusing collection of health disorders that reads like a laundry list of today's malaises. The list includes:

- Muscle spasms
- Joint pain
- Skin and connective tissue tenderness
- Numbness
- Tingling in the hands or feet
- Difficulty sleeping
- Debilitating fatigue
- Anxiety
- Headaches
- Difficulty verbally identifying objects
- Digestive problems

- Sensitivity to weather and temperature changes
- Circulatory problems
- Upper respiratory problems
- Premenstrual syndrome
- Frequent or chronic infections
- Food allergies
- Depression
- Trouble concentrating—"brain fog"

You needn't experience all the above symptoms to have fibromyalgia. Most people experience only a few distressing symptoms at a time, with the type and severity of symptoms changing over time.

In order to meet the American College of Rheumatology criteria for fibromyalgia, you must have BOTH of these symptoms:

- History of widespread pain, on both sides of the body, both above and below the waist, present for at least three months; this must include pain in the neck, chest, and upper or lower back.
- Pain upon palpation in at least 11 of 18 "tender point" sites. No one knows why these 18 points on the body are characteristically tender to touch, but all people with fibromyalgia will at some time experience tenderness at a minimum of 11 sites.

(For more information about diagnosing fibromyalgia, see Chapter 3.)

PAIN IN FIBROMYALGIA

While the type and severity of symptoms vary from person to person, there's one thing that every man, woman, and child with fibromyalgia shares in common: pain.

Each person experiences the pain of fibromyalgia differently. Some describe shooting, knifelike, or stabbing sensations; others call it throbbing, cramping, aching, or burning. Pain may stay in about the same place, or move from one part of the body to another, and vary in intensity according to the time of day, your activity level, the weather, how much sleep you are getting, and the degree of stress in your life. And your pain may come and go: Just when you feel you can't stand it anymore and decide to see a physician, suddenly you feel better.

Most fibromyalgia pain is felt in the muscles, although pain around the joints may also occur. Less frequently, the joints themselves may feel painful, although joint destruction, such as that seen in arthritis, does not typically occur in fibromyalgia. Headache pain is also common.

Beyond making you feel bad, pain has physical consequences. Research shows, for example, that chronic pain can suppress the immune system, leaving you more vulnerable to colds and infections. It can chronically raise blood pressure, boosting the odds of heart attack and stroke. And chronic pain may even encourage the growth of some types of cancer. Chronic pain doesn't just feel bad; it's truly bad for your health.

TENDER POINT PAIN

In addition to widespread, chronic pain, people with fibromyalgia also feel pain at specific, localized tender points. Tender points are distinct areas of the body that feel painful when pressed. Tender points may or may not hurt at other times, but are significantly painful when touched with a moderate degree of pressure—enough pressure to whiten your nail if you press down with your thumb.

Over the years, various researchers have identified hundreds of tender points on the bodies of people with fibromyalgia. Based on studies, the American College of Rheumatology has chosen 18 of these points upon which to base the defining diagnosis of fibromyalgia. People without fibromyalgia express only minor discomfort when these 18 points are pressed; those with fibromyalgia, however, experience intense, white-hot pain upon palpation of at least 11 of these 18 sites. Tender points are located at the base of the skull, above and between the shoulder blades, below the elbows, in the lower back, on the hips, and behind the knees. (See diagram.)

Tender point pain can also be found in other disorders, such as tendinitis. But in fibromyalgia, tender points are located on *both* sides of the body and cannot be traced to injury or overuse. And when touched, they generally do not send or "refer" pain elsewhere in the body as is the case with other pain disorders, such as myofascial pain syndrome.

BACK AND NECK PAIN

People with fibromyalgia complain about pain in the neck and back. It's not clear if pain in the neck and back

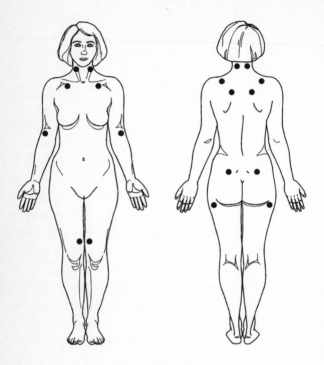

In order to make a diagnosis of fibromyalgia, doctors look for pain upon palpation in at least 11 of 18 identified "tender point" sites.

ILLUSTRATION ADAPTED BY CHUCK CHEZOSKY.

is a triggering event leading to the development of fibromyalgia, or if the neck and back are common sites for fibromyalgia pain once the condition has developed—or both.

Back pain is extremely common in the general population. Some people attribute this to our upright walking position, which puts a lot of weight and pressure on the lower spine and supporting muscles. Others argue that back pain is largely a physical manifestation of a psychological reaction to internalized anger and stress. Whatever the underlying reasons, back pain is the number one cause of disability in this country. So we shouldn't be too surprised that it affects people with fibromyalgia, too.

You may experience back pain on one or both sides of the body, high or low or in between. Most of the time, you will be able to tell that the pain is in your muscles, not in the joints. You may be fooled into thinking the joint is involved, however, because sometimes the structures around the joints, called tendons and ligaments, are involved in fibromyalgia. But usually this discomfort can be distinguished from true pain in the joint itself. It's important to determine the source of the pain because problems with the joints in the back are managed quite differently than muscle pain.

People with fibromyalgia experience neck pain from chronically tense neck muscles, which cause the bones in the neck to lose their natural curve and puts pressure on the nerves between the bones. Neck muscle tension is very painful; pain due to pressure on the nerves can be excruciating.

HEADACHE PAIN

Headaches in fibromyalgia are often described as migraine-like, sometimes accompanied by nausea and/or sensitivity to light. Or you may experience tension headaches, with a sensation of tightness or pressure like a tight band around the head or over one section of the head, such as the temples, across the forehead, or radiating up the neck or down into the shoulders. Like migraines, fibromyalgia headaches may not respond to over-the-counter pain relievers.

Headaches may also be related to another condition frequently found in people with fibromyalgia: temporomandibular joint disorder (TMJD). The temporomandibular joint is a highly complex mechanism located where the lower jaw meets the skull. Perhaps because of poorly fitting joint components or problems with the muscles or ligaments surrounding the joint, TMJD can cause a lot of pain in the joint itself, in the face, or the jaw, and may also produce headaches.

FATIGUE AND POOR SLEEP

Although everyone feels tired on occasion, the ongoing exhaustion often associated with fibromyalgia takes the word *fatigue* to a whole new dimension. Your fatigue may be moderate at times, or so severe that even simple tasks like getting dressed or brushing your teeth seem daunting. You may feel tired or drained after very mild activity, such as cooking dinner, or too tired to fold clothes or walk to the mailbox. Crushing fatigue can impact your performance at work, starting long before your workday ends—perhaps as soon as you get out of bed in the morning.

The debilitating fatigue often seen with fibromyalgia may very well be the result of chronic sleep deprivation (among other possible causes). Many people with fibromyalgia can fall asleep without difficulty, but then fail to reach a deep state of restful and restorative sleep essential for good health. Instead, they sleep lightly in a kind of "twilight state," tossing and turning, awakening at the slightest sound. In the morning, rather than feeling rested and refreshed, they get out of bed exhausted.

DEPRESSION AND ANXIETY

Changes in mood and emotional state are common in fibromyalgia, sometimes progressing to depression and/or anxiety. Who wouldn't feel depressed or anxious when living with constant pain, life-changing fatigue, and lousy sleep? Lack of sleep, night after night, is enough in and of itself to make you depressed. In fact, studies have shown that depression and other symptoms of fibromyalgia can be induced in people without the disorder simply by depriving them of sleep for about three days!

Some researchers believe there may be a biochemical link between fibromyalgia and depression or anxiety. Even if you aren't among the 25 percent of people with fibromyalgia who meet the criteria for clinical depression, you may understandably feel "blue" or "down" about your condition and its impact on your life. Of course, any feeling of depression or anxiety can further interfere with activities at work and at home.

IRRITABLE BOWEL SYNDROME

Studies on people with fibromyalgia show that up to 70 percent may experience irritable bowel syndrome. This may manifest alternately as diarrhea and constipation, abdominal pain and gas, nausea, and painful gut contractions. You may feel an "urge to go" but be unable to move your bowels when you try. Sometimes irritable bowel syndrome symptoms can be severe enough to keep you housebound, never knowing when symptoms will start. Your symptoms may lead your physician to mistakenly diagnose your condition as colitis or Crohn's disease, both diseases of the intestine associated with cramping, diarrhea, and sometimes blood in the stool.

GASTROESOPHAGEAL REFLUX DISEASE (GERD)

People with fibromyalgia may also experience gastroesophageal reflux disease, abbreviated GERD. In this disorder, partially digested food, instead of passing through the stomach into the small intestine, backs up into the esophagus (the tube leading from the mouth to the stomach), which gets "burned" by the acidic stomach material. Some people call this heartburn. GERD may progress to the point where the delicate tissues of the esophagus and throat become eroded and eating is unpleasant. Chronic GERD may sometimes cause a sore throat, can trigger asthma, and even increases the risk of cancer of the esophagus.

MORNING STIFFNESS

Many people normally feel a bit stiff when they first wake up. After a few minutes, the stiffness usually disappears and they're ready to start the day. But people with fibromyalgia may continue to feel stiff more than 30 minutes after rising. They describe their joints as feeling "glued down" or "jelled." The stiffness is usually extensive, affecting all parts of the body, and in some cases, persisting throughout the day.

PARESTHESIA

People with fibromyalgia sometimes experience a feeling of tingling, numbness, or swelling in the hands, arms, feet, or legs, although no swelling actually exists. Such a feeling is called a paresthesia and may occur at more than one place on the body at a time. Paresthesias may be especially apparent upon rising and often occurs along with morning stiffness. Although bothersome, paresthesias are not harmful and generally needn't limit your activities. On the other hand, there may be serious underlying medical problems (such as diabetes, autoimmune disease, or thyroid disease) causing the paresthesias. For this reason, it is appropriate to do screening blood tests to rule out a serious underlying condition when paresthesias are present.

CIRCULATORY PROBLEMS

Many people with fibromyalgia have poor circulation. Their fingers feel cold and turn pale, perhaps even blue, when exposed to cold winter temperatures or summer air conditioning. Less often, the same thing may happen to toes. Sometimes the color changes are accompanied by pain. The problem, called Raynaud's disease, is a circulatory disorder that makes the hands and sometimes feet hypersensitive to cold. Raynaud's phenomenon can occur by itself or may be triggered by fibromyalgia or another underlying illness.

People with fibromyalgia can sometimes be sensitive to cold and heat without experiencing Raynaud's phenomenon. Some malfunction in the circulatory system seems to be involved.

MUSCLE TWITCHING

Perhaps you've experienced a phenomenon where you're just about to fall asleep when one of your legs suddenly jerks involuntarily. The jerk may be so sudden and intense that it even wakes you up. For some people with fibromyalgia, the twitching continues throughout the night. You feel like you simply must move your legs or you'll never get comfortable. This condition, called restless legs syndrome, is especially common in fibromyalgia.

Occasionally, restless legs syndrome can even be painful, but more often its most bothersome aspect is that it prevents you from falling asleep or it repeatedly wakes you up. People with fibromyalgia already have enough trouble sleeping soundly; restless legs syndrome just makes matters worse.

DRYNESS

The inside of the mouth, the lining of the nose, and the eyes are supposed to be moist. Wetness provided by saliva or tears serves many purposes, including trapping potentially harmful bacteria. People with fibromyalgia sometimes suffer from Sjogren's syndrome, an autoimmune illness in which the secretions to the eyes, nose, and mouth are reduced or eliminated. In addition to being uncomfortable, the excessive dryness of Sjogren's syndrome can increase the risk of infection in these areas.

PELVIC PAIN

Women with fibromyalgia may have unusually painful menstrual cramping, irritable bladder syndrome, or other pelvic pain. Women with irritable bladder syndrome need to urinate frequently, feel pressure in their lower abdomen, and may experience incontinence.

NAME YOUR SYMPTOM

In addition to all their other symptoms, people with fibromyalgia may also suffer from:

- Unexplained visual problems
- Auditory dysfunction
- Respiratory difficulties
- Allergies
- Hypersensitivity to environmental pollutants

If you have fibromyalgia, you may have other symptoms to add to this list. Because research is ongoing for this disorder and its causes are still under investigation, it's possible that many of your unexplained symptoms may be related to fibromyalgia. You may have observed some symptoms worsen under certain conditions. Lack of exercise, too much exercise, changes in the weather, major stressful events in your life, premenstrual syndrome, or infections such as a cold or flu, can bring on symptoms or make existing symptoms worse. Symptoms may also vary due to one or more *other* health problems that may occur *along with* fibromyalgia. Some of the other conditions share similar signs and symptoms and can either be misdiagnosed as fibromyalgia or can coexist with fibromyalgia. The long list includes:

- Attention deficit disorder, with or without hyperactivity
- Candida overgrowth (yeast infections)
- Carpal tunnel syndrome
- Chronic fatigue syndrome (CFIDS, CFS)
- Cognitive problems
- Costochondritis
- Depression
- Digestive problems
- Eating disorders
- Fever
- Gastroesophageal reflux disease (GERD)
- Gulf War syndrome (GWS)
- Hair and nail problems
- Headaches and migraines
- Hearing problems
- Hepatitis
- HIV/AIDS
- Hypoglycemia

- Hypothyroidism
- Immune system weakness or immune dysfunction
- Irritable bladder (urethral syndrome)
- Irritable bowel syndrome (IBS)
- Joint pain
- Lupus
- Lyme disease
- Mitral valve prolapse
- Multiple chemical sensitivity
- Myofascial pain syndrome (MPS)
- Osteoarthritis
- Polymyalgia rheumatica
- Post-polio syndrome
- Premenstrual syndrome (PMS)
- Raynaud's disease
- Rheumatoid arthritis
- Seasonal affective disorder (SAD)
- Sexual dysfunction
- Sjogren's syndrome
- Sleep apnea
- Sleep dysfunction
- Sore throat
- Swollen lymph nodes
- Temporomandibular joint disorder (TMJD)
- Vertigo
- Weight gain

Of these, let's take a closer look at rheumatoid arthritis, chronic fatigue syndrome, Lyme disease, HIV infection, myofascial pain syndrome, and candida overgrowth.

RHEUMATOID ARTHRITIS

Fibromyalgia is considered to be a rheumatic disease, which is any disease characterized by pain and stiffness of the muscles, tendons, or joints. Many people with fibromyalgia are cared for by rheumatologists, medical doctors specializing in rheumatic disorders. Men and women with other rheumatic diseases, such as rheumatoid arthritis or lupus, are at greater risk for developing fibromyalgia. In fact, about 20 percent of people with rheumatoid arthritis will develop fibromyalgia. So having one rheumatic disease not only doesn't protect you from getting another, it may actually predispose you to it.

CHRONIC FATIGUE SYNDROME

Fibromyalgia may occur with, or be confused with, chronic fatigue syndrome (CFS). The conditions are similar in so many respects that some clinicians argue that they are both points on the same line, with fibromyalgia anchoring the point at which muscle aches and pain predominate, and CFS anchoring the point at which fatigue predominates.

There are important differences between CFS and fibromyalgia, however. In CFS the lymph nodes in the neck and armpits may be sore and tender, and a sore throat may be present. People with CFS have histories of extreme exhaustion lasting at least six months, which is not usually the case with fibromyalgia, unless the person has both CFS and fibromyalgia. (For more information about how to distinguish between fibromyalgia and CFS, see the section in Chapter 3.)

LYME DISEASE

Lyme disease may also mimic fibromyalgia. Following the bite of an infected deer tick, a person will usually develop a specific type of rash and flu-like symptoms, followed by muscle aches and pains that may be similar to fibromyalgia. Or true fibromyalgia may develop following the infection. If you suspect you have fibromyalgia but the symptoms have come on fairly suddenly, ask your doctor to rule out Lyme disease. Lyme disease usually responds well to early, intensive treatment with antibiotics, and may be prevented by a vaccine.

HIV INFECTION AND AIDS

Although research is still sketchy, early studies indicate there may be something in either the treatment or progression of HIV infection that causes fibromyalgia-like symptoms to develop. Dr. Gregory Gardner of the University of Washington, Seattle, found 8 percent of the HIV-positive patients surveyed met the criteria for fibromyalgia. Other studies estimate 10 to 29 percent of HIV-positive patients exhibit fibromyalgia-like symptoms. More research is needed to explore and explain this correlation.

MYOFASCIAL PAIN SYNDROME

Another condition frequently seen with fibromyalgia—and sometimes confused with it—is myofascial pain syndrome (MPS). Myofascial pain syndrome is different than fibromyalgia because instead of painful tender points, people with MPS have "trigger points." These are hard, lumpy areas in the muscle, which, when pressed, *refer pain* to other regions of the body. In contrast, pressing on tender points causes intense *localized* pain that stays in place. While not the norm, some truly unfortunate people are burdened with both fibromyalgia and MPS, making their lives a near-constant pain experience.

CANDIDA

Although routinely overlooked, chronic yeast infections throughout the body often occur with fibromyalgia. Candida infections may perpetuate the tender points, as do all infections, because the body's defenses are busy fighting the bad guys. When large amounts of circulating antibodies attach to the candida antigen, they can form immune complexes which build up or accumulate in the tissues. This can cause a "serum sickness" type of reaction that causes many of the symptoms associated with fibromyalgia. Fibromyalgia patients with histories of chronic vaginal yeast infections, thrush, digestive problems, regular use of antibiotics or steroids, or sensory hypersensitivity may also be suffering from candida overgrowth. Because the symptoms of candida may overlap with those of fibromyalgia, this common condition may go undiagnosed.

Candida infections can cause bloating, abdominal upset, and muscle pain and aches in some people. Treatment with an anti-yeast agent can drastically improve symptoms; however, it may *increase* symptoms (in the short run) as the yeast organisms are destroyed.

CHILDREN AND FIBROMYALGIA

Children can also suffer from fibromyalgia, referred to as juvenile primary fibromyalgia syndrome (JPFS). Little research has been conducted since Dr. Muhammad Yunus first identified JPFS in 1985. We do know that children suffer many of the same symptoms as adults: widespread pain, fatigue, nonrestful sleep, headaches, stiffness, numbness, swelling of the fingers and hands, irritable bowel, and/or frequent urination. Interestingly, more boys suffer JPFS than girls, for some unknown reason.

In children as with adults, stress often triggers the onset of fibromyalgia. A number of recent studies indicate that fibromyalgia may run in families, suggesting there may be a genetic component to the disorder. Other studies link fibromyalgia in children with prior sexual, emotional, or physical abuse. A Finnish study found that children with JPFS are at higher than average risk for depression and recommended that the depression be treated along with the JPFS.

Correct diagnosis is just as important for children as it is for adults. A 1996 study done in Italy reported that 1.2 percent of students, grades 3 to 12, who answered a questionnaire met the criteria for JPFS. Given that 7 percent of all pediatric office visits are related to musculoskeletal complaints, JPFS is probably missed or misdiagnosed more often than it is properly identified. Physicians may confuse JPFS with Lyme disease, juvenile rheumatoid arthritis, hysteria, tendinitis, inflammatory arthritis, low back pain, hypothyroidism, or reflex sympathetic dystrophy.

When a child repeatedly complains of chronic pain, parents and guardians need to be wary of the catchall diagnosis of "growing pains" or psychological problems. Trust your child and pursue an accurate diagnosis.

HOW DID THIS HAPPEN TO ME?

No one knows exactly what causes fibromyalgia, but scientists have collected a trail of possible clues, including:

GENETICS

Genetics may play a role in fibromyalgia because the condition tends to run in families. (Some researchers have suggested that may only be because it's such a common disorder.) No specific gene or hereditary link has been identified, but research continues in this area. In any case, if you have a relative who has experienced the widespread muscle pain and fatigue of fibromyalgia, along with some of its other symptoms, you may be at greater risk for developing the disorder yourself. Even if your relative has never been formally diagnosed with fibromyalgia, you may notice similar symptoms.

One study on genetics and fibromyalgia suggests the disorder may be passed on to children by an "autosomal dominant" mechanism. If true, that means about half of all children who have one parent with fibromyalgia can expect to develop fibromyalgia themselves. More genetics studies are needed to clearly establish this mechanism for inheritance.

SENSITIVITY AMPLIFICATION

Sensitivity amplification is sometimes referred to as the "irritable everything" syndrome. Our survival depends on being sensitive to things in the environment: noise, light, touch, taste, and movement. But with a sensitivity amplification, you overreact to these things. In fact, your reaction can be so intense it can feel overwhelming. For example, some people with fibromyalgia simply cannot tolerate the buzzing sound of fluorescent lights. They must escape from the irritating noise and can think of little else until they do.

In fibromyalgia, nerve endings become hypersensitive, causing the brain to interpret some stimulation as pain that might not be considered pain by people without fibromyalgia. Chronic overstimulation may be responsible for some of the chronic pain of fibromyalgia.

ABERRANT MUSCLE COMMUNICATION

Muscles normally communicate and coordinate with each other via our nervous system, indicating their position and degree of contraction by the action of certain neurotransmitters (chemicals released by the nervous system). This helps us be aware of our body's position and helps us gauge how much muscle strength is needed for a particular task, such as crossing our legs.

People with fibromyalgia have aberrant or faulty muscle communication because they lack the proper sensory feedback. Instead of working in tandem with the neurotransmitters, the muscles have to rely on being able to "feel" their own activity accurately. This can make it quite a challenge to perform simple tasks such as drinking a glass of water or picking up a ringing telephone. It can be done, but it just takes practice. Muscles may contract beyond what is needed for the task.

TRIGGERING EVENTS

Some people with fibromyalgia say their syndrome began after a triggering event, such as a car accident, severe flu, childbirth, or a death in the family. Certainly many people experience stressful events without developing fibromyalgia. Perhaps some people have an underlying predisposition to the disorder that is somehow "turned on" in a stressful situation. Such stressors may also cause existing fibromyalgia to suddenly get worse, often referred to as a flare or flare-up.

DYSFUNCTIONAL NEUROTRANSMITTERS

Neurotransmitters are the body's chemical messengers, transmitting information within the nervous system (the brain and spinal cord), as well as between the nervous system and the rest of the body. Neurotransmitters help control many bodily functions, including sleep, pain, mood, and muscle function.

Low levels of the neurotransmitter serotonin have been implicated in many disorders, including depression and anxiety. The body uses serotonin and other neurotransmitters to control muscle function, pain sensations, sleep cycles, and the immune system. Some researchers have found that people with fibromyalgia are significantly deficient in serotonin. It is not clear whether low serotonin is a possible cause of fibromyalgia or a result.

Another neurotransmitter, called Substance P, is responsible for transmitting painful impulses to the brain and spinal cord. It also produces a nerve-generated response that dilates blood vessels. In addition, Substance P can cause fluid and proteins to migrate from inside the cells to outside the cells. In people with fibromyalgia, levels of Substance P are sometimes as much as three times higher than normal. This may explain the generalized pain sensations and the feeling of swelling sometimes experienced by people with fibromyalgia.

It is interesting to note that serotonin and Substance P work together. In fact, serotonin regulates the amount of Substance P in our bodies. Too little serotonin in the body results in too much Substance P. Dr. I. John Russell, associate professor of medicine/clinical immunology at the University of Texas Health Science Center at San Antonio, says, "The elevated Substance P in fibromyalgia is the most dramatically abnormal laboratory measure yet documented in these patients." Clearly, the regulation of neurotransmitters plays a major role in the severity of fibromyalgia. Again, we don't know if it's a cause or a result.

Two other neurotransmitters, epinephrine and norepinephrine, which are involved in the body's preparation for "fight or flight," help regulate heart rate, blood pressure, and rate of breathing. Constant release of these neurotransmitters is thought to be one outcome of chronic stress, leading to elevated blood pressure and possibly fibromyalgia.

Growth hormone may be depressed in people with fibromyalgia. Growth hormone is secreted by the brain during a particular phase of sleep and is used by the body to maintain normal muscle metabolism and repair.

The hormones cortisol, DHEA, and thyrotropin-releasing hormone have also been implicated in fibromyalgia. These chemicals are related to the complex interaction between the brain, pituitary gland, adrenal glands, and thyroid gland and help control fundamental functions like metabolic rate and cellular growth and development.

IMMUNE DYSFUNCTION

The immune system appears to function abnormally in fibromyalgia. The immune system is a complex group of cells and chemicals that work together to protect your body from infection. Researchers have found that some elements of the immune system do not function properly in people with fibromyalgia. For example, the immune system's "natural killer cells" are less active against bacteria in people with fibromyalgia. Natural killer cells are a vital first-line defense against cold, flu, and infection.

Another immune system component called cytokines have been found to be either too high or too low in fibromyalgia. And unexpected immune reactive proteins have been found in the skin of people with fibromyalgia. These proteins form only when the body is mounting an immune reaction to an invader. Their presence indicates yet another possible immune dysfunction associated with fibromyalgia.

SAME PAIN, DIFFERENT NAMES:
A BRIEF HISTORY OF FIBROMYALGIA

Symptoms of muscle aches and body pains have been described throughout history. In the Bible (Job 30:17), Job laments, "The night racks my bones, and the pain that gnaws me takes no rest." Alfred Nobel, who invented dynamite and originated the Nobel Prize, may have endured fibromyalgia, too. Many letters to his mistress describe multiple muscle aches and pains, migraine headaches, gastrointestinal disturbances, cold intolerance, and problems when the weather changed.

Tender points were first described in 1816 by Scottish physician William Balfour. In the years that followed, the medical community gave the disorder many names, including chronic rheumatism, pressure point syndrome, and myalgia. In the late 1800s, a psychiatrist wrote about neurasthenia, a condition characterized by fatigue, muscle aches and pains, and psychological disturbances.

The term "fibrositis" was coined in the early 1900s to describe the sore spots found in patients with muscular rheumatism. But for decades, the diagnosis of fibrositis, with its vague definition and lack of a clear, identifiable cause, unsettled many clinicians, who often considered the diagnosis to be invalid. Throughout the twentieth century, while modern medicine made great strides in understanding and treating all sorts of diseases, fibrositis languished in a kind of medical limbo, rarely studied, little understood, and often dismissed as a "catchall" for vague complaints of unknown origin.

Finally, in 1987, the American Medical Association recognized fibromyalgia as a legitimate illness, largely because of a study by Dr. Don Goldenberg published in the *Journal of the American Medical Association (JAMA)*, which described the symptoms, lab findings, and treatment results of 118 patients with fibromyalgia. Goldenberg used the terms *fibrositis* and *fibromyalgia* interchangeably at the beginning of the paper; then he switched exclusively to *fibromyalgia* through the rest of the paper.

In another *JAMA* article, Dr. Robert Bennett wrote: "The term *fibromyalgia* has evolved from another with the same meaning, namely, fibrositis." The later term, Bennett argued, was a misnomer and not accurate. "Itis" implies inflammation. Muscle biopsies of patients with fibromyalgia typically do not show evidence of inflammation, and the pain of fibromyalgia usually does not respond well to anti-inflammatory medications. "Myalgia," on the other hand, refers to pain of the muscles without implying inflammation. Myalgia is therefore a more appropriate term to use.

On January 1, 1993, the Copenhagen Declaration established fibromyalgia as an official disease recognized by the World Health Organization. The document described the condition as painful, non-articular (not in the joints), and predominantly involving the muscles. The World Health Organization added several other symptoms to the list, including "the presence of unexplained widespread pain or aching, persistent fatigue, generalized morning stiffness, and non-refreshing sleep." The

Copenhagen Declaration also recognized depression and anxiety as possible manifestations of the syndrome, and declared the problem to be the most common cause of chronic, widespread musculoskeletal pain.

After decades of being snubbed by mainstream medicine, the collection of symptoms we now call fibromyalgia went from being a questionable diagnosis to *the world's most common cause of chronic, widespread musculoskeletal pain.* In terms of official medical recognition, fibromyalgia has arrived—and so has the funding for further medical research.

RESEARCH ON FIBROMYALGIA

Now that fibromyalgia has been recognized as a distinct disease entity by the World Health Organization and the American College of Rheumatology, more physicians and researchers have become interested in studying it. In 1999 the National Institutes of Health spent $4.7 million on fibromyalgia research, up from $3.1 million in 1998, and three times the funding provided in 1993.

Research aimed at uncovering the cause(s) of fibromyalgia, as well as to developing treatments and perhaps even a cure, is currently conducted or overseen by:

- National Institute of Neurological Disorders and Stroke (NINDS)
- National Institute of Nursing (NINR)
- National Center of Complementary and Alternative Medicine (NCCAM)

- National Institute of Arthritis and Musculoskeletal and Skin Diseases (NIAMS)

Fibromyalgia research seeks to answer several key questions and address specific symptoms, particularly:

EFFECTIVE PAIN RELIEF

Chronic pain is one of the most debilitating symptoms of fibromyalgia. Unremitting pain is implicated in the development of mood disorders, including depression and anxiety. Many current fibromyalgia studies focus on the use of non-sedating, non-narcotic, or non-addictive medications to relieve pain. Sometimes low doses of two medicines are used in combination to boost their pain relief properties while reducing the side effects associated with higher doses of one medicine alone.

UNDERLYING PROBLEMS CAUSING A HEIGHTENED PERCEPTION OF PAIN

Abnormal levels of several chemicals in the body, including Substance P and nerve growth factor (NGF), are involved in the heightened perception of widespread pain. The Substance P level is often three times higher than normal in people with fibromyalgia. NGF is often about four times higher than normal. Researchers are studying how these two chemicals produce the perception of pain, and how they interact with one another. It is possible, for example, that excessive NGF is the underlying cause of elevated Substance P. Perhaps medications or other interventions that inhibit NGF or Substance P will relieve pain.

Abnormal Nervous System Interactions

One theory on the basic cause of fibromyalgia suggests that the autonomic nervous system (which controls breathing, heart rate, and other basic body processes) may be under-responsive. Low levels of a cortisol and growth hormone, and high levels of Substance P and NGF, all indicate this may be so. One area of current research focuses on cytokines, a group of messengers that regulate the immune system. The possible connection between cytokines and fibromyalgia may help explain why some people develop fibromyalgia following an infection.

Abnormal Serotonin

The neurotransmitter serotonin plays a number of roles in the body, including regulating sleep cycles, mood, and pain perception. Researchers are continuing to investigate how abnormal levels of serotonin may contribute to fibromyalgia.

Other areas of fibromyalgia research overlap with studies of other conditions, especially chronic fatigue syndrome, myofascial pain syndrome, and autoimmune diseases such as rheumatoid arthritis.

You Can Make a Difference

Research is ultimately our best hope for developing better treatments and finding a cure for fibromyalgia. As you take charge of your individual treatment plan, ask yourself if you'd like to be part of the bigger solution. If you live near a teaching hospital or an affiliate hospital that is investigating fibromyalgia, you may wish to participate in a research study.

To find out where studies are taking place, contact the American Fibromyalgia Syndrome Association, 6380 E. Tanque Verde, Suite D, Tucson, AZ 85715. Call 520-733-1570, or visit their Web site at *www.afsafund.org*.

As a study participant, you probably will not know whether you are receiving an active drug or a placebo, whether your CT scans show an abnormality, for example, or much about the methods being used. Some people find the role of "guinea pig" disconcerting at best. At worst, you could be denied a promising new therapy or drug because you have been selected as part of a control group.

On the positive side, by your participation, you'll be directly helping to advance knowledge about a condition that you know from personal experience can be enormously debilitating. You could be helping spare others what you have endured, perhaps a child with her whole life still in front of her. As a study participant, you may receive effective new therapies before the rest of the world, or at least be in a good position to hear about them first. Who knows? Your study could be the one that helps researchers put this painful puzzle together, finds a cure, and ends the suffering for people with fibromyalgia.

2

Finding Your Own Road to Relief— An Integrative Approach

If you or someone you know suffers from fibromyalgia, chances are your most pressing issue as you read this book is how to get *immediate and long-term relief*. I wish I could give you a quick and simple way to escape the chronic pain, severe fatigue, and other distressing symptoms of fibromyalgia, but the truth is there is no easy way, no magic pill that works for everyone.

To find the relief you're looking for, you're going to have to do some work. You're going to have to dig for information that applies to your unique situation, piece together what works best for your changing symptoms, and create your own evolving path to recovery.

My goal for this book is to make your task as easy as possible by providing you with all the information I give my own patients and pointing you in the direction of dozens of conventional and complementary resources for further help and support. In Chapter 1, I laid out the scope of the problems we face with fibromyalgia. In the rest of the book, I'll provide detailed information on what to do about it—how to diagnose possible underlying causes of fibromyalgia and how to sort through your various treatment options for taming the wide variety of symptoms that characterize this chronic illness.

Before diving deep into all the nitty-gritty details, let's first get an overview of what it takes to cope successfully with fibromyalgia. When embarking on any journey, it helps to have a road map. In this chapter we discuss:

- Knowing what you're up against
- Listening to your body
- Building a team
- Turning down pain
- Getting the sleep you desperately need
- Living the good life again

KNOWING WHAT YOU'RE UP AGAINST

At the time of this writing, no one knows what causes fibromyalgia, nor is there agreement on the best way to treat it. In time, as research continues and our understanding grows, all that will change. But for now, our limited knowledge makes it necessary to treat the *symptoms* of fibromyalgia when no underlying cause has been identified. Compounding this problem, many people with fibromyalgia also suffer from one or more other health problems (see Chapter 1). Many of these conditions are plenty challenging on their own. Potential combinations of health issues can make your diagnosis more tricky and your treatment more complicated.

You must get used to the idea that fibromyalgia relief is not going to be "one-stop shopping." Studies show a multidisciplinary approach to symptom management is more effective. My own experience has taught me that by integrating the most effective tools from conventional and complementary/alternative medicine, people with fibromyalgia **can** live more comfortable and productive lives.

The best way to start your journey is with a positive, winning attitude. *Expect to feel better*. And expect to *take charge* of making that happen. Gather lots of information: read books, clip articles, talk to people with personal and professional experience, stalk health food stores, and surf the Internet. (For a list of Web sites and other resources, check the listing at the back of the book.) Keep your eyes and ears open for new information and new clues in this ongoing mystery.

Under the guidance of your conventional physician, your CAM practitioner, and other experienced health professionals, *try different approaches*. Work with your health care providers to triage your treatment plan, starting with the simplest, gentlest, least invasive treatments. Pay attention to what works, monitor the results, and move on to the next option if what you're trying fails to work. Failure simply provides another piece of vital information for you and your health care team. Remember, the more failures you experience, the closer you are to figuring out what will succeed.

Don't get discouraged! Fibromyalgia is tough, but so are you. If it helps, think of yourself as a scientist, a warrior, or an explorer on a mission of discovery. Yes, you're part of a team, but you can't find your own path to relief by turning your fate entirely over to others. Avoid the trap of feeling like a passive victim; take charge of your health and healing. Know what you're up against and know that, with the right help, you have what it takes to win.

LISTENING TO YOUR BODY

Your first vital step to easing the symptoms of fibromyalgia is to become acutely aware of your physical self—your body and its signals. While it's true that the right lab tests, at the right time, interpreted by the right professionals, can be very important for diagnostic and treatment purposes (see the section in Chapter 3), nothing takes the place of direct self-knowledge through ongoing personal experience.

Unfortunately, many successful adults and even some children lead lives that have systematically trained them to ignore their bodies. Overachievers are particularly at risk for "body ignorance"—often not realizing when it's time to stop working or playing to eat, drink water, or rest. Many people just do not pay close enough attention to their physical needs and sensations. When illness occurs, symptoms have to get fairly intense before they are noticed. With a chronic illness like fibromyalgia, this is a prescription for trouble. The longer it takes you to notice your body's signals, the more difficult it becomes to dial down those symptoms and get effective relief. Fibromyalgia is not an ailment for which you can simply pop a pill and get on with your life. Successful management of fibromyalgia demands you pay attention to yourself.

Certainly no one would ask for this illness. But if you have it, use the opportunity to practice more self-awareness and self-care. One useful way to pay closer attention to your body and its signals is to keep a symptom diary. Even if you feel well-tuned to yourself and your body, keeping a daily diary can help you keep track of changes (and perhaps patterns) in your pain, fatigue, and other symptoms in relation to:

- Time of day
- Season
- Weather
- Emotional or physical stress
- Type of food you've recently eaten
- Household chores you've recently performed
- Work
- Exercise and other activities

When keeping a symptom diary, you may learn, for example, that you feel worse after eating a heavy meal but feel better after talking to a dear friend or walking in the fresh air. Once on paper, some of these correlations may seem obvious, but until you consciously think about them, you may be missing some important clues as to what triggers or relieves your symptoms. Other connections may be more subtle and easier to miss unless you force yourself to pay attention. Carefully monitoring the *early* stages of muscle tension, for example, can be especially useful for people with fibromyalgia.

It doesn't take much time to keep track of how you're feeling throughout your day. Just jot down a few notes, making sure you indicate any connections you notice, even if they seem unlikely. Over time, patterns may emerge that could provide your health care team with important information to guide diagnosis and track the effectiveness of various treatments.

BUILDING A TEAM

Equally important on your road to relief is forming a collaborative partnership with a competent physician who has significant experience with fibromyalgia. This could be your family practitioner, internist, or rheumatologist. He or she will take a careful and detailed history, order appropriate diagnostic tests, and help oversee and coordinate your ongoing treatment. Under the guidance and with the knowledge of this physician, you may need to try many different therapies, both conventional (see the section in Chapter 3) and complementary/alternative (see the sections in Chapters 7 to 12), before discovering what works for you and putting it all together (see Chapter 13).

You may need to "shop around" a bit to find a doctor who has the conventional medical experience you need *and* is open to collaborating with you and with other professionals, such as a nutritionist, a physical therapist, an herbalist, a massage therapist, and an acupuncturist. Even if your primary physician is not knowledgeable enough to refer you to these or other practitioners, he or she should at least be open to the idea of your working with other experts and should be willing to hear what they might have to offer. If not, find someone who is.

Remember, it's not a personal insult to your regular doctor if you search for someone more experienced with fibromyalgia. After all, you wouldn't go to a plumber to fix your car, no matter how good the job he did on your bathroom last year. You have a right to choose what you need, when you need it. (See the section in Chapter 3 for more information about finding and working with a conventional physician.)

TURNING DOWN PAIN

In the midst of so many varying symptoms and so many possible causes, those who endure fibromyalgia inevitably share a single, common bond: pain—the kind of pain that keeps on hurting day after day, year after year.

As we discussed in Chapter 1, fibromyalgia pain comes in two varieties: widespread, chronic pain and focused, tender point pain. While tender point pain is far from pleasant, many people with fibromyalgia find the widespread, chronic pain to be the most debilitating. Unlike the useful, focused pain of an acute health problem (like a toothache), which motivates you to protect the painful area and seek immediate help, the dispersed, chronic pain of fibromyalgia serves no protective function. In fact, it can actually work against your efforts to get well. In time, the endless pain of fibromyalgia can bring a kind of invisible, creeping fog over one's world, little by little eroding stamina, hampering productivity, and draining the joy from life.

Regardless of your other symptoms, the number one objective of most people with fibromyalgia is immediate and long-term pain management. While you may never get rid of *all* the pain, a personalized treatment plan can greatly lessen your discomfort, and in some areas, even eliminate it. Winning the battle against pain requires better understanding, so you can ease the pain that responds to treatment and learn to live better with the pain that doesn't.

Pain is both emotional and physical, both subjective and objective. Only you know where you hurt, how much you hurt, and what, if anything, helps. Of course, you can try to describe your pain to others, but only you really know what you're talking about. You may use common words like cramping, stabbing, or twisting, but the listener can only understand these in terms of his or her own experiences, not yours.

Our subjective perception of pain varies widely, depending on our personalities and our immediate thoughts and feelings. For instance, stress—like losing a job, ending a relationship, or worrying about a problem—can leave you temporarily less tolerant to pain. Further complicating the picture, living with chronic pain can wear you down emotionally, contributing to both depression and anxiety—either of which can, in turn, further magnify the perception of pain.

But the subjective and emotional nature of pain does not negate its objective, physical reality. Research shows that some people are genetically predisposed to experience more pain than others. Feelings of pain result from chemical events inside nerve cells in the body and brain. These changes in chemistry inside our nerve cells alert us to pain by releasing a neurotransmitter called Substance P (see Chapter 1). *People with fibromyalgia have three times more Substance P than those without the disorder.* And those who smoke and have fibromyalgia experience even higher levels of this neurotransmitter.

Researchers now think that these abnormally high levels of Substance P are partially responsible for the chronic pain suffered by many people with fibromyalgia. Over time, heightened pain can become a backdrop to life, like a constant "white noise" felt within the body. Many people respond unconsciously to this irritation by slightly but continuously contracting their muscles, especially those in the back and neck. Chronically tensed muscles have the unfortunate effect of further heightening muscle pain, creating an escalating cycle of pain.

EASING MUSCLE TENSION AND PAIN

The key to coping with the pain of fibromyalgia is to not let it escalate. Anything that relaxes the muscles and keeps them relaxed is helpful. Sooner is better than later. Once pain escalates, it's harder to control without outside help. Biochemical interventions (herbs, medications, etc.), structural interventions (massage, spinal adjustments, etc.), or mind–body interventions (relaxation techniques, biofeedback, etc.) may be needed.

You can avoid the risks and expense of more invasive treatments by soothing muscle tension before it builds.

- Play close attention to your posture: how you hold your head, how you stand, sit, and lie in bed. Be especially kind to your overworked neck. According to experts, for every inch you hold your head too far forward, the weight of your head doubles! Poor posture and stress both tend to jut your head forward, and holding your head too far forward causes more stress. Is it any wonder your neck, shoulders, back, and jaw hurt? (For more posture tips, see Chapter 6.)

- Think about how you move through space. Try not to lean; stay upright and balanced. Practice walking as if you are being held up by an imaginary string coming out of the top of your head. Walk and stand tall. The Alexander technique is an example of a movement therapy that helps correct poor posture and dysfunctional patterns of movement which tend to perpetuate muscular pains.

- Throughout the day (set your watch, if it helps), consciously relax your muscles. Sit or lie comfortably, and beginning at one end of your body (say, your feet), systematically relax your muscles. Pay special attention to your neck, shoulders, and face. Then stand up straight, lower your shoulders, open your mouth slightly, and let your face "hang" from your head without moving your head forward. (If you can't relax your facial muscles easily, try faking a smile—it takes far fewer muscles to smile than frown, and you'll look nicer, too!)

- Several times a day, take deep, slow breaths through your nose and exhale through your mouth. Breathe slowly; don't hyperventilate.

- Avoid exposure to cold temperatures and abrupt changes of temperature, like going in and out of air-conditioned rooms, which may cause muscles to contract. Warm, dry weather is less aggravating to muscles and joints than cold, damp weather. Dress warmly. Have a jacket ready when going into air conditioning. Try to avoid sleeping in air-conditioned rooms. And avoid outdoor activities during the hottest hours of summer.

- Get moving. Gentle to moderate exercise—when started *slowly* and increased *gradually*—increases circulation, improves flexibility, releases pain-killing endorphins, and gives your tense muscles something to do with all that tension! I'm not suggesting you jump into an advanced aerobics class, but it's not wise to avoid exercise entirely just because your muscles hurt. An individualized exercise program designed with your specific needs in mind can take the edge off pain and boost your health in many important ways.

Swimming (especially in a heated pool) and walking are excellent for many people. (You'll find more information on exercise in Chapter 6.)

- Apply heat or cold for 15 to 20 minutes. Heat helps increase blood flow and relaxes muscles. Cold numbs pain and reduces inflammation and swelling. When using heat or cold to treat your muscle pain, remember the following safety tips:

  - Apply heat or cold only to healthy, unbroken skin.
  - Place a towel or padding between you and your source of heat or cold to protect your skin from burning or freezing.
  - After treatment, check the area for discoloration or swelling.
  - Moist heat works best. Use a warm, wet towel or a moist heating pad (the sponge type). A baby's clean disposable diaper soaked with hot water will stay warmer longer than a wet towel, plus the plastic liner will keep your clothes or bedding dry. Warm baths, showers, and whirlpools can provide great relief.
  - Cold packs, crushed ice in a plastic bag, or even a package of frozen peas wrapped in a cloth are safer and can be used longer than plain ice applied directly to the skin. If you use direct ice, rub it quickly back and forth over the skin for no longer than five minutes to avoid skin damage.

Rub Out Pain with Massage

Sore muscles like to be touched and rubbed. You can massage yourself at home, or get a family member or friend to assist you. If you'd like to try self-massage, first take a bath or use a heating pad to relax your muscles. Put some lotion or oil on your hands and massage the sore area using a circular motion. Massage oils allow the hands to glide over sore muscles more easily. Special creams developed for pain relief, available in drugstores, might prove helpful as well. Hand-held electric massage devices can also be used (but not on sensitive joint areas!) to assist with self-massage. These devices provide pleasant, vibrating sensations that loosen muscles and offer temporary, superficial relief. Don't expect them to do more than they are intended to do, however. They are not a substitute for a skilled massage therapist.

If you're too tired for self-massage or your hands hurt too much, perhaps a relative or friend would be willing to give it a try. Family members, who sometimes feel powerless in the face of your fibromyalgia, may enjoy an opportunity to help you feel better. There are many good manuals available for learning massage techniques.

Another option is to hire a massage or bodywork therapist who's experienced with fibromyalgia. A massage therapist who is overly aggressive could trigger a major flare-up of fibromyalgia symptoms. Whether you do self-massage or a family member, friend, or professional massage therapist works with you, the key to avoiding a setback is to start out cautiously, using gentle techniques.

There are many types of massage therapy (see the section in Chapter 10). Some may be new to you. For example, craniosacral release (CSR) can ease pain by normalizing the flow of spinal fluid within the area surrounding the brain and spinal cord. The more traditional massage kneads the muscles and connective tissue, boosting circulation and releasing pain-relieving endorphins. Not all massage and bodywork therapies are well suited for every health problem. Take the time to learn about each modality and discuss your options with your physician before starting any treatments.

EASING HEADACHES

Headache pain may be due to excessive or chronic muscle tension, or to other problems, such as poor posture, eyestrain, stress, injuries, food allergies/sensitivities, chemical sensitivities, sinus infections, dental problems, or even genetics (you can actually inherit a tendency for headaches). Whatever the cause, headaches are a nuisance that can adversely affect your overall well-being. Some headaches, such as migraines, can be totally incapacitating.

People who get frequent headaches may have lower levels of the brain chemical serotonin and greater blood vessel reactivity (the blood vessels contract and expand more than normal). An article in the November/December 1993 issue of the medical journal *Headache* linked tension and migraine headaches to an abnormally high level of Substance P. This may explain why people who live with fibromyalgia are also prone to headaches.

Many people rush to treat all headache pain with over-the-counter drugs, such as ibuprofen or aspirin. I caution against relying on these drugs as your first line of action. All medications put an added burden on the liver and kidneys and can cause side effects. Among other risks, overuse of pain medications can cause rebound headaches.

Before reaching for a pill, there are plenty of self-directed measures to try. Here are some simple yet effective strategies for relieving tension headaches:

- Relax in a comfortable chair or bed to keep muscles from tensing up. Darken the room if possible and close your eyes for five minutes while you breathe deeply and slowly. Visualize the pain leaving your body each time you exhale.
- Drink a caffeinated beverage, but don't overdo it. While a moderate amount of caffeine can reduce headache pain, too much may aggravate the problem.
- Wrap a blue-ice gel pack in a towel and place it on your head where the pain is greatest.

COPING WITH "FLARES"

Fibromyalgia pain that suddenly worsens is called a flare. Although flares may seem to come when you least expect them, they are almost always the result of additional stress of some kind. These are called triggers—specific events or activities, big or small, that for any number of reasons create just enough stress to suddenly escalate the pain cycle.

The trigger could be as minor as rolling over in bed, or as major as losing a loved one. More often, it's something in between, like jet lag, poor sleep, a cold, or too much exercise. Situations that would have little effect on people without fibromyalgia can harshly impact someone with this illness. A major stressor—like moving, losing your job, or a physical injury—can really throw you for a loop. Even "good stress"—like getting married—can trigger a flare, especially if sleep, meals, and other routines are disrupted. Even treatments can cause a flare, such as taking a medication to treat a yeast infection, which can cause a "die-off" reaction as toxins are released, leaving you feeling ill for a few days.

You can save yourself from experiencing significant pain and misery by nipping flares before they get out of hand, or at least by being prepared for them at the first sign. Here's where that symptom diary discussed earlier can really pay off. Signs of an impending flare include:

- Fasciculations—small twitches caused by groups of muscles that fire randomly. These jerks and spasms indicate muscle or nerve irritation. Before a flare, these twitches often get worse.
- You may drop things more than usual and feel weaker than usual. Your muscles are becoming unreliable as they try to limit the force of their contractions to keep you below the pain threshold.
- One hand or foot may feel colder than the other due to abnormal blood vessel constriction.

- You may feel dizzy when changing positions, or you may misjudge your location in space and bump into furniture or fall over curbs.
- You may have difficulty judging the weight of items.
- You may spill food while eating.
- Fibro-fog (the inability to think clearly) can descend. You may not remember things that happened yesterday, or even just hours ago. You may even be unaware of being in a flare.
- Depression may worsen.

Minimizing Flares

You can't always prevent flares, but with awareness and knowledge, you can minimize their frequency and severity. Go easy on yourself; don't compare your reactions to stress with that of other people, and don't underestimate your potential vulnerability. Avoid unnecessary changes in your routines and practice healthy lifestyle behaviors (see Chapter 6).

If you feel you may be on the brink, mobilize your family and/or supporters. Let them know what might happen and what to look for during a flare so they can help you. Ask for help. In asking, you give people who want to help you a chance to do something useful. Depending on your relationships, ask different people for different types of help. Ask for meals or for groceries to be delivered to your door. To minimize the need for shopping during a flare, keep staples and nonperishable items on hand, plus a supply of portion-sized cooked meals in the freezer. Ask others to drive so you don't have to. Ask for company, if it helps.

Simplify your life and dial down your physical and emotional stress as much as possible. Find creative ways to do less. Consider, for example, automatic payments of as many bills as possible so you don't have to write checks.

Don't sweat the small stuff. Skip the wash if you have clothes for tomorrow. Let the toys lay around in the living room; it really is no big deal. Break big problems down into tiny, manageable chunks and deal with one piece at a time. Make a list of the negative elements in your life. Decide which ones you can change and which ones you cannot. Focus on changing what you can, step by step. Ignore or accept what you can't change.

Give yourself plenty of quiet time. Stay home when you can. Be as lazy as you can get away with; sleep as much as you can, whenever you can. Baby yourself. Remind yourself there will be better times ahead.

While in the middle of a flare, respect your pain. I know that may sound odd, but pain is a powerful force: Don't fight it; you can't win. In time, it will pass. Lower your expectations and ride it out.

MEDICATIONS IN MODERATION

If, after trying a number of strategies for dealing with the chronic discomfort of fibromyalgia, your pain has not significantly improved, or it has escalated into a flare, you and your physician may wish to explore pain medications. Some doctors are in the habit of rushing ahead and quickly prescribing what I think ought to be "Plan B" in pain management: drugs.

If there were a magic pill to get rid of your fibromyalgia, believe me, I'd suggest you go get it right now. But it's not that simple. Medications work only to varying and limited degrees. And all medications—*all of them*—carry risks and potential side effects.

Nonetheless, there comes a time when turning to medications makes sense. The first thing to keep in mind when trying a new medication is that it may not work. You may need to try several different drugs or even a combination of drugs before you find the medication or medications that help your pain with the fewest, most tolerable side effects. Don't expect a medicine that works well for one person to work equally well for you. People with fibromyalgia often experience unusual responses to medicines. For example, a medicine that produces sleepiness in most people may keep someone with fibromyalgia awake. The best strategy is a "try it and see" approach.

Never take a medication without a full discussion with *your* physician. Only trained health professionals can recommend proper dosages and discuss risks and benefits in the context of *your* particular situation. In Chapter 3, I discuss several medications that have a better-than-average risk–benefit ratio.

GETTING THE SLEEP YOU DESPERATELY NEED

Because lack of restful sleep can bring on fibromyalgia-like pain in people without fibromyalgia, some researchers have suggested that fibromyalgia pain is largely due to ongoing sleep disturbances. While we now know there's more to it than that, chronic sleep problems certainly do make pain, fatigue, and other fibromyalgia symptoms worse.

People with fibromyalgia report two kinds of sleep problems. They may fall asleep quickly but wake too early (3:00 to 5:00 A.M.), exhausted but unable to go back to sleep. Or they take a long time to fall asleep, toss and turn most of the night, and then drag themselves out of bed as late as possible in the morning, feeling exhausted.

Although there's no surefire way to improve your sleep, and what works for Jane may not work for Sally, here are some suggestions worth trying:

- Routines are important, just as they were in childhood. Develop a routine you can follow nightly.
- Before you begin your nightly routine, make a list of things you'd like to accomplish the following day. Be realistic about your goals. Put the list where you can find it easily and then put it out of your mind.
- Artificial lighting can confuse your internal clock. About an hour before bedtime, dim the lights in your home. This will reduce your energy level and promote rest.
- Take a warm bath, meditate, or do relaxation exercises right before bedtime.
- Limit or eliminate caffeine, alcohol, cigarettes, and cigars. All can keep you awake.

CREATING A RESTFUL ROOM

Set up your bedroom or sleeping area in such a way that you immediately feel relaxed whenever you walk in the room. Soft colors, low light, and comfortable decor work well for most people. Close closet doors and get rid of clutter. Put computers, books, and paperwork in another room where they can't "nag" you to think about them. Block out light with room-darkening window shades and buy a pair of sleep shades for your eyes. Eliminate as much noise as possible. If necessary, use soft foam earplugs (found at hardware stores) or keep a radio on nearby, turned to an easy listening or classical music station. Keep the volume very low.

Sleep on a mattress that's right for you. Most people with fibromyalgia prefer a mattress that is soft on top with a firm foundation below. Invest in a high-quality pillowtop mattress, waterbed, or air-chamber bed. Many stores will let you try one at home for 30 days and will refund your money if it's not right for you.

Use a comfortable pillow. There's no steadfast rule for this. Some like down pillows; others are allergic to them. You need neck support, so be sure your pillow can mold into a shape that allows your neck to relax. The only way to find a pillow that's right for you is to test some out. The Comfort-U™ total body support pillow is a product developed for fibromyalgia sufferers that may be worth trying.

MEDICATIONS FOR SLEEP

Conventional medicine often relies on the use of medications. Some doctors make a diagnosis and immediately prescribe a drug to treat the disorder. I prefer a less-is-more progression based on an integrative approach that employs the useful tools and techniques of CAM with the technical prowess of Western medicine. This provides a wider range of treatment options. I find also that by involving patients in their own treatment, their heightened sense of empowerment and control enhances the effectiveness of any therapy.

Sleep problems can often be solved without drugs. When all else fails, or when the individual simply cannot bear another nonrestful night's sleep, the occasional use of sleep medications may be helpful. For some people, ongoing use of an antidepressant medication may improve the quality and quantity of sleep. The potential risks and benefits of an antidepressants and other medications are discussed in more detail in Chapter 3.

LIVING THE GOOD LIFE AGAIN

Despite the chronic pain, fatigue, headaches, and other symptoms of fibromyalgia, with the right attitude, information, professional help, and personal support, you *can* live the good life again. If you are currently missing one of these key healing ingredients, now is the time to do something to change that.

Before you get caught up in all the details of your specific diagnosis and treatment options, here are some tips for creating a solid foundation upon which to build your new, healthier, happier life:

- **Develop a positive, healing attitude.** You are entitled to a good and healthy life, and you have what it takes to learn how to cope well with fibromyalgia and anything else life throws your way. When talking to others or talking to yourself, stop using words and phrases that reinforce illness and start talking like someone who's on the mend. For example, instead of making general, negative statements like "I'm sick of being so tired" or "This pain is really killing me," try being more specific and positive (or at least neutral) by saying, "Today is a good day to relax more" or "This pain is really talking to me today." When feeling especially down or discouraged, take one small step toward learning more about your problem or trying a new approach. Any action, no matter how small, will help. Even in the midst of deep depression, a part of you can say to yourself, "Wow, I'm really depressed today. What is one small action I can take today to feel better?" If you can't think of anything, you can always call a friend or a support group (check the resource listing) for an idea, or just to talk.

- **Information is power.** Don't wait passively for information to find you; actively hunt it down wherever you can. Read books and articles, ask lots of questions, take notes, surf the Net, listen actively during doctor visits. You don't have to go get a degree in medical research, but learn what you can and stay informed. No matter how many health care professionals you employ to help you, ultimately *you* are in charge. Don't travel blind.

- **Get professional help.** You may be the captain of your ship, but you need a lot of experienced hands on deck if you want to get anywhere without sinking. First and foremost, you need a first mate—a competent physician with plenty of experience in diagnosing and treating fibromyalgia. Doctors who ignore the problem, or who only recently got interested in the diagnosis, can't provide the expertise and guidance you need. Keep looking and interviewing until you find the right partner.

- **Ask for personal support.** Chronic illness can be lonely. Some of us are lucky enough to have lots of personal support; the rest of us have to reach out and get it. If you don't have family members or friends who actively support and encourage you, get some! Ask people you already know to consider helping and supporting you more. They may not realize what you are going through and how much you need them now. If they don't respond as hoped, make new friends at local support group meetings or by regularly telephoning other people with fibromyalgia. (For information on how to reach others with fibromyalgia, see the resource listings.) It's easier to forgive your loved ones for falling a bit short when you have other support within your reach.

HELPING CHILDREN COPE WITH FIBROMYALGIA

As difficult as it can be for adults to cope with fibromyalgia, for children the condition can be even more devastating. Chronic pain and fatigue can put a black cloud on childhood, lowering self-esteem and leaving children feeling powerless. They have so little choice or control over their lives as it is.

Children look to the adults in their lives to set the tone for how to cope with adversity. Be as positive as possible and get help immediately. Studies indicate the earlier fibromyalgia is diagnosed, the better chance there is for significant resolution. In the largest study to date, symptoms abated in 73 percent of children within two years of diagnosis.

Once a diagnosis has been made, parents or primary caregivers need to sit down with the child, explain what's happening, and present a plan of action. Set guidelines on how the child will deal with school, teachers, school-mates, and extracurricular activities. Help your child learn some easy stress management skills, and assure him or her that there is a network of loving, supportive people who can and will help along the way. Encourage close relationships with health care providers to foster trust. Above all, let your child know you'll do everything you can to help. Here are some helpful suggestions:

- **Be honest.** Answer questions as honestly as possible, but don't say more than you need to for her or his age.

- **Be proactive at school.** Most children spend more time at school than anywhere else, so this is where most lifestyle changes must be implemented. Make an appointment with the teacher and the principal to alert them to your child's condition and ask for their cooperation. Schools must, by law, make accommodations for children with disabilities. Be sure your child has two sets of books, if possible—one to keep at home and one at school. This will minimize or eliminate the need to lug heavy books back and forth each day. Give your child a backpack to carry homework. Try to arrange for rest times or extra minutes between classes in the higher grades. It's wise to find a simple explanation to give to your child's playmates, as well. They deserve to know what's going on with their friend, and once they understand something about the disorder, they may even take an active role in maintaining your child's well-being.

- **Get family counseling.** Chronic illness affects every member of the family, not just the patient. Don't wait until you have serious relationship problems. Invest in a few sessions of "preventive maintenance" now.

- **Let them be kids.** No parent wants to see his or her child suffer. But you can't keep your son or daughter in a bubble, cut off from the world. Though it may sometimes go against your better judgment, make a conscious effort to let your child be a kid. Sure, there will be times when doing so will have adverse effects. But in the long run, it will probably do more psychological harm to keep him confined and severely limited.

- **Stay positive.** Focus on the good. Watch your language. Give lots of hugs and smiles. If you need to express negative emotions related to your child's condition, do it away from the child, with an understanding adult.

The future for children diagnosed with fibromyalgia is bright. They can benefit from most of the suggestions and strategies found in this book, and they will certainly reap the rewards of any medical progress. With your love and support, plus the support of a caring health care team, your child can cope with this challenge and blossom.

3

Finding the Right Physician, Getting Diagnosed, and Sorting Out Your Treatment Options

Now that we've looked at the scope of the fibromyalgia problem in Chapter 1, and an overview of your various relief options in Chapter 2, it's time to focus more specifically on how to find and work with a competent, cooperative conventional physician—your essential "first mate" on your journey to greater comfort and better health.

To be honest, many of my fellow physicians are still in the habit of acting like *they* are in charge of your voyage. For years, conventional medical doctors have been systematically trained to treat patients like passive, naive children. They've gotten used to making many important decisions with little discussion about options and alternatives. They're just not used to treating the patient like a valuable, active member of their medical team.

Of course, in the last 15 years we've seen dramatic changes in the expectations and interests of patients, who increasingly see themselves not as victims waiting passively to be healed, but as informed consumers actively pursuing health. With this change has come growing public interest in alternative medicine and various healthy lifestyle strategies, such as nutrition and exercise. As baby boomers continue to age (reluctantly), they are no longer content to be simply disease-free; they want optimal health and are pursuing it with a passion—and with their pocketbooks.

Conservative by nature, conventional medicine typically ignores the passing winds of popular change. But with consumers now spending more than $27 billion on complementary/alternative health approaches, even the steadfast American Medical Association has had to wake up and smell the herbal tea.

Many doctors who only a year or two ago turned a blind eye to CAM are now willing to consider its many potential benefits. In the long run that's good news because, in my view, the merging of conventional and CAM approaches into integrative medicine provides a new, more powerful level of patient care than either can offer on its own.

For people with fibromyalgia and other chronic illnesses, the evolution toward integrative medicine means greater recognition, more accurate diagnosis, and many more treatment options. If you have fibromyalgia, your chances of being told "it's all in your head" are still higher than I'd like, but not as high as before.

On the down side, there are now a growing number of doctors who use the term "fibromyalgia" as a catchall for all sorts of other problems they can't immediately diagnose. I've heard rheumatologists complain that they are seeing patients who have no business being in their offices because they don't have fibromyalgia but some other disorder causing similar symptoms. Today we have a wide range of physicians who, at one end of the spectrum, still refuse to acknowledge the legitimacy of fibromyalgia, and at the other extreme, use the diagnosis as a "garbage can" label for a collection of other disorders.

What this means to you, the savvy medical consumer, is the age-old adage: *buyer beware*. Be wary. Be informed. Do your homework, ask lots of questions, and be the captain of your own ship—but not without that trusty first mate. Trying to diagnose and treat fibromyalgia on your own, without the guidance of the right doctor, is a bad idea that, sooner or later, will not serve you well. In this chapter, I tell you what to look for in a conventional physician, what questions to ask, and how to get the best care.

FINDING THE BEST CONVENTIONAL PHYSICIAN FOR YOU

It is absolutely essential to your successful diagnosis, treatment, recovery, and long-term well-being to find the right physician *for you*—someone who is medically competent, experienced with fibromyalgia, knowledgeable in or at least open to CAM, and easy to talk to. In my opinion, you really can't skimp on any one of these four requirements.

If you're lucky, your current medical doctor already fits the bill. But the odds are you're going to have to shop around. You can start your search by contacting some of the support organizations in the resource listing. Almost all of them have Web sites, so it's easy to contact them via the Internet. Telephone calls and letters work fine, too. National organizations can put you in contact with local chapters. Go to a local chapter meeting or call a few members and ask for referrals to physicians in your area who are experienced with fibromyalgia. Sometimes local physicians may even be members themselves.

You could also contact the American College of Rheumatology (see the resource listing). Rheumatologists specialize in the treatment of disorders characterized by pain and stiffness, including fibromyalgia.

Don't settle for one referral; collect a few and make appointments. Simply explain to the receptionist that you are interested in meeting with the doctor for a few minutes to get to know him or her better, and that you're not coming in for a full consultation or treatment. Most physicians do not charge for this type of visit.

WHAT MAKES A GREAT DOCTOR?

A great doctor is a great partner. He or she is technically prepared to help you manage your fibromyalgia and philosophically prepared to work with you and various additional health care professionals, as you see fit. Given that fibromyalgia is a chronic disease, you will likely be dealing with your physician for years to come. Don't just settle for someone conveniently located down the street.

Take the time to find someone truly up to the job. Here's what to look for:

Technical Competence

- *Institutional endorsement*: Did she or he graduate at the top of the class or at the bottom?
- *Peer endorsement*: Within the medical/complementary medicine communities, the names of the more respected practitioners keep coming up again and again.
- *Patient endorsement*: Word-of-mouth recommendations are sometimes the most reliable source of information.
- *Experience*: Is fibromyalgia a "sideline" or a focus of the practice? For how long? What results has the physician had in treating other fibromyalgia patients or those with similar disorders?

Balanced Philosophy

- *Collaborative approach*: Is the physician comfortable working with you and with other practitioners as partners in a team? Does she or he recognize the value of using both conventional and complementary/alternative therapies? If not, there's no need to go any further.
- *Communication*: Is the physician comfortable talking with other medical doctors or CAM practitioners, sending them progress and consultation notes regarding shared patients?

- *Recognition of limitations*: Ask the physician what disorders or symptoms she or he is not comfortable treating. If the answer is none, this should be a warning. No one practitioner or discipline can successfully treat all conditions.

The bottom line is to find someone you can trust. Beyond technical competence and a balanced philosophy, your doctor ought to be the type of person you could tell the most personal, perhaps even embarrassing, things when necessary for your proper diagnosis or appropriate treatment. Your physician needn't be your best buddy. But you should have the feeling that you can count on him or her to stick with you for the long haul and go the extra mile for you.

CULTIVATING THE TEAM APPROACH TO COLLABORATIVE CARE

Once you've found the right physician, the next step is to begin cultivating a team approach to collaborative care. Both you and your physician have specific responsibilities to the team. In addition, your physician has the responsibility of communicating with your other health care professionals.

YOUR RIGHTS AS A PATIENT

As a health care consumer, you have certain rights, including:

- The right to ask for help
- The right to be treated as a person, not merely a "fibromyalgia case"

- The right to be informed and educated about your condition
- The right to be listened to regarding your needs and concerns
- The right to receive quality medical care
- The right to be involved in medical decisions that affect you

Don't abdicate any of your rights to your doctor or anyone else. Exercising your rights as a patient is more important to your health than you may think. Studies show that a positive, active role in treatment may actually speed the healing process.

YOUR RESPONSIBILITIES AS A PATIENT

In addition to your rights as a patient, you also have important responsibilities. Sometimes, it seems like it would be nice to just sit back and let someone else take care of everything, especially when you're not feeling well. But being a grown-up with a mysterious chronic illness calls for action. Responsibilities confer power and control. When you meet your responsibilities, you maximize your power in a situation; you've done your part.

You can get the most for your time and money when you:

- Provide accurate information about your medical history, current and past medications, and current symptoms. To be concise and complete, it helps to write down as much of this information as possible *before* your first visit. Even if you expect to fill out questionnaires in the office, bring your notes.

- Inform your doctor of any side effects you may be experiencing as a result of medications you're taking.
- Inform yourself about your condition (you're already taking this step by reading this book).
- Keep track of symptoms and be prepared to give your doctor a list of any changes in your appetite, diet, weight, sleep patterns, sexual interest, ability to concentrate, memory, and bowel/urinary habits.
- Let your doctor know of any recent stressful situation such as divorce, death of a loved one, family problems, or job-related changes.
- Actively participate in your own treatment. Ask questions, no matter how trivial they may seem to you.
- Follow through on therapies to the best of your ability. No therapy will work if it isn't implemented.
- Honestly express your concerns, feelings, and fears to your physician.

Remember, *you* are the one who ultimately decides what diagnostic tests to accept and what treatments to pursue. You have that right, but along with it comes the responsibility to communicate to your doctor the results of all tests and all decisions to start, alter, or discontinue treatment.

A VISIT TO YOUR PHYSICIAN

Once you have selected a physician and are clear about your rights and responsibilities, it's time for your initial consultation. If you have a condition that requires immediate attention—like an adverse reaction to medication—do not wait for your scheduled appointment. Promptly go to an urgent care facility or hospital emergency room and get help. Conventional Western medicine is unrivaled in the treatment of emergency conditions.

Before you go to your scheduled office visit, ask yourself a few questions: What is the main reason I'm going to the doctor today? What are the three main questions or issues I want to talk with my doctor about? What else worries me about my health? What do I expect my doctor to do for me today?

Your time with the doctor will likely be limited, so make a list (in order of importance) of the problems you wish to discuss. Identify the three most pressing problems or concerns and ask about them right away, at the beginning of the visit, before time runs out. Write down the answers, including the names of new medicines or changes in the dosage or timing of medicines you might already be taking.

If there are specific treatments or therapies you've heard or read about for the symptoms of fibromyalgia, ask your doctor about them. He or she will tell you if such treatments are likely to be beneficial for your symptoms. If you require a prescription, ask for one now.

You can maximize the effectiveness of your office visit or telephone consultation by keeping the following in mind:

- Don't expect a cure for fibromyalgia. There isn't one—yet.
- Don't expect hand-holding. Use a support group, friend, or family member for that.
- Don't waste time on irrelevant small talk.
- Have specific questions *in writing* ready for the doctor.
- Repeat back what you hear to avoid misunderstanding.

During your visit, if you don't understand the doctor's instructions or why therapies are being changed, ask for clarification. Sometimes an appointment goes by so fast and the information is so complex that it's easy to become confused. Ask questions! The only stupid question is the one not asked. The more information you gather, the more helpful a team member you can be.

STALKING THE ELUSIVE (CORRECT) DIAGNOSIS

As many fellow fibromyalgia sufferers will attest, getting the right diagnosis is far from quick and easy. The unfortunate truth is, most people with fibromyalgia have the disorder for an average of four or five years before being properly diagnosed! In addition to four or five years of chronic pain, poor sleep, bowel problems, headaches, and other associated problems, many also are forced to put up with not really knowing what's wrong with them.

Some people also develop depression, perhaps in part because there seems to be so little hope or help.

Thanks in large measure to the World Health Organization, the National Institutes of Health, and the American College of Rheumatology, fibromyalgia is now recognized as a "real" disorder. But there's a certain amount of lag time between the official recognition of a disorder by major health organizations and its practical recognition by individual physicians. Perhaps you have already encountered one or more doctors who aren't quite up to speed on this illness. If so, try to put that frustration behind you. Now that you have found someone with experience with fibromyalgia, you can finally get the help you deserve.

It's important to keep in mind that fibromyalgia is really not a diagnosis in the truest sense of the word. *Diagnosis* comes from the Greek *dia* (to divide into two parts or distinguish between) and *gnosis* (knowledge or understanding). *Webster's Dictionary* defines diagnosis as "the art or act of recognizing the presence of disease from its signs or symptoms and also deciding as to its character." Without understanding the underlying cause of the problem, the term fibromyalgia is merely a label for a collection of symptoms. That said, we will call it a diagnosis anyway, because that's what most people call it.

CORRECTLY DIAGNOSING FIBROMYALGIA

With so many people going so long without an accurate diagnosis, you'd think fibromyalgia was terribly difficult to identify. Actually, in less than 10 minutes, an experienced rheumatologist or other trained physician can apply pressure to specific points on the body and determine if you have fibromyalgia.

To review, the American College of Rheumatology's criteria for fibromyalgia are straightforward. You must have *both* of the following conditions:

- History of widespread pain, on *both* sides of the body, *both* above and below the waist, present for at least three months; this must include pain in the neck, chest, and upper or lower back.
- Pain upon palpation in *at least* 11 of 18 tender point sites.

But, as you know by now, the health issues associated with fibromyalgia go far beyond body pain. The only way to fully and correctly diagnose and treat someone with fibromyalgia is to also look for and treat their other underlying conditions. Conventional medicine prefers to deal with isolated disorders. But like it or not, diagnosing and treating fibromyalgia often requires diagnosing and treating one or more of the following underlying or coexisting conditions:

- Sleep apnea
- Hormone dysfunction
- Drug side effects
- Malabsorption
- Poor biomechanics and posture

- Allergies
- Rheumatoid arthritis
- Candida overgrowth
- Multiple chemical sensitivities
- Chronic infections
- Exposure to environmental pollutants and toxins
- Anger
- Anxiety
- Depression
- Frustration
- Energy imbalances

LABORATORY TESTS

Strictly speaking, you don't need a lab test to identify fibromyalgia. But as I've pointed out, fibromyalgia often does not arise in and of itself, without other health problems. To assist in diagnosis, your physician may order one or more laboratory tests, including:

CBC

The letters stand for "complete blood count." This test counts the number of all the different types of blood cells in your blood sample, including red blood cells, white blood cells, and platelets. Aberrant values for any of these might indicate one of many possible conditions. In conjunction with the CBC, your physician might also order a chemistry panel, which is used to assess the functioning of your kidneys and liver, and looks at the amount of cholesterol and other chemicals in the blood.

Thyroid Tests

The thyroid gland produces hormones that regulate metabolism. Thyroid dysfunction is relatively common as we age. If the levels of thyroid hormones are too low, the pituitary produces too much thyroid-stimulating hormone (TSH), and the result can be some of the same symptoms as seen with fibromyalgia. Thyroid hormone levels may also be too high, in which case the pituitary reduces the output of TSH. I think the thyroid tests deserve a closer look.

The most commonly ordered thyroid test measures TSH level. There are two thyroid hormones: T3 and T4. T4 is the less active of the two. It is produced by the thyroid gland and then converted to T3 outside the gland. T3 is three to four times more potent than T4. Blood tests of T3 and T4 measure how much of these hormones in the blood are bound to carrier proteins. When bound to proteins, they aren't available to stimulate metabolic activity in the cells, and so this test may not reveal much. A T7 level screening test measures the amount of free T4. "Free" hormones are looking for action, which is what we like to see. A measure of all of the above is included in the typical "thyroid function panel."

Free T3 is not usually included in most thyroid function panels. This exclusion can lead to misleading test results. Free T3 measures the amount of unattached T3 (the most active form of thyroid hormone) that is available to actually do something. If a person gets back normal test results, she or he could still have a low free T3, which means T4 is not adequately converting to T3.

The patient could have a condition sometimes referred to as Wilson's syndrome, which most physicians have never heard of. (Another kind of Wilson's syndrome—a genetic disorder of copper metabolism that has nothing to do with the thyroid—is better known.)

If your doctor wants to test your thyroid function, ask him or her to include a measure of your *free T3*.

Adrenal Tests

The adrenal glands are found just above your kidneys on either side of your spine. Like the thyroid gland, they produce hormones that control body functions. Some of them are very important in the body's response to stress. In diagnosing fibromyalgia, I check DHEA-sulfate level, as well as a cortisol level. DHEA is a hormone produced by the adrenal gland that is used as a building block for a number of other hormones. People with a low DHEA level are often tired and achy, and they have difficulty concentrating.

An elevated cortisol level can be caused by stress or, very rarely, by an adrenal tumor. An elevated level is associated with lower immunity and sometimes an elevated sugar level. "Adrenal exhaustion" is the term for an adrenal gland that isn't meeting the demands placed on it. This diagnosis is not yet recognized by the medical establishment.

Autoimmune Tests

In autoimmune diseases, the immune system mistakes the body's own cells as foreign invaders that need to be destroyed. Rheumatoid arthritis and lupus erythematosus are considered to be autoimmune disorders, at least in part. When the body turns against itself it produces characteristic antibodies, specialized immune chemicals that help in the attack process. Fibromyalgia sometimes occurs together with autoimmune disease, and some of its symptoms may mimic these disorders. These tests help determine if an autoimmune disease is present and perhaps playing a role in your fibromyalgia symptoms.

An arthritis panel is typically included in these tests. It usually includes a uric acid level (screening for gout), an ANA (antinuclear antibodies) measure, a rheumatoid factor (for rheumatoid arthritis), an ASO titer (antistreptolysin O is an antibody produced against strep infections—sometimes anti-strep antibodies can cross-react with joint tissues, thus leading to joint aches), an ESR (erythrocyte sedimentation rate), and a CRP (C-reactive protein). The last two are nonspecific markers of inflammation. If any of these results are abnormal, further testing is warranted.

Candida Overgrowth Tests

Candida albicans is a type of yeast that can cause problems for people with fibromyalgia and other disorders. Although the yeast is found in many places and in many people, it doesn't usually cause problems unless something enables it to grow rapidly. Then it produces a very unpleasant infection of the mouth, the gut, the skin, or the vagina. Candida tests include those looking for antibodies against the yeast, a sign that the yeast organism is out of control. The diagnosis (and treatment) of candida overgrowth is controversial and not accepted by most of the medical community. This controversy could be resolved by performing a couple of well designed studies.

Food Allergy Tests

It's possible that some of the symptoms you're experiencing are due to food allergies or sensitivities, or that food allergies may be one result of fibromyalgia. (see Chapter 5 for a discussion of this issue.)

Infectious Disease Tests

Several infectious diseases may cause some of the same symptoms as fibromyalgia. These include Lyme disease, HIV infection, syphilis, herpes virus infection, and others. Before jumping to a diagnosis of fibromyalgia, your doctor may want to make sure you don't have an active infectious illness.

Sex Hormone Tests

Abnormal levels of sex hormones could be causing some of your problems. Your physician may measure levels of estrogen and progesterone (for women) and testosterone (for both men and women).

Stool Analysis

A stool analysis can reveal problems with malabsorption, bacterial infection, parasites, yeast overgrowth, bowel organism imbalances, and "leaky gut syndrome" (a disorder sometimes seen in patients with fibromyalgia, in which food molecules are absorbed intact instead of fully digested, causing myriad problems).

Hair Analysis

Chemical tests on samples of your hair can reveal heavy metal exposure or poisoning. This could be relevant if you work around or with metals (iron, aluminum, etc.), live in an area where the water is not treated for metals, or if your home was built before 1978, when lead was banned from housepaint. If hair analysis shows lead or other toxins, blood and possibly urine tests are warranted. If the blood or urine tests are also abnormal, then environmental tests of your home, water, or workplace may be needed.

Hypercoagulability Tests

Hypercoagulability is a term used to describe an abnormal thickening of blood. In some patients with symptoms of fibromyalgia, the blood is not thick enough to produce dangerous clots, but it can adversely affect the circulation of blood oxygen and other nutrients to tissues. Poor circulation due to hypercoagulation can cause fingers and toes to become cold, numb, or turn blue—symptoms often associated with fibromyalgia.

More Tests

After your physician reviews the results of your tests, some tests may be repeated, or different tests may be ordered. Ask for explanations of your test results, and be sure to *get copies of all lab tests* for your own files. This will help you keep track of what's been done and when. And if you later want to see another practitioner, you'll avoid wasting time and money on needless retesting.

Diagnosing Sleep Problems

Sleep disturbances are common in fibromyalgia and may be due to many possible causes. Some people have difficulty getting a good night's rest because of sleep apnea, a condition in which you stop breathing for a short period during sleep, followed by a gasp for air. Each time your breathing momentarily stops, your brain rouses you from sleep just enough to get your breathing restarted, often without your awareness. The cycle continues through the night, resulting in exhaustion from a lack of deep (delta wave) sleep.

A significant number of people who have been told they have fibromyalgia actually have undiagnosed sleep apnea. To screen for this condition, you can do nocturnal pulse oximetry. This test is usually provided free of charge or at low cost by home oxygen supply companies. It is a noninvasive test done in the privacy of your home. If the results show an abnormality, a sleep study in a sleep laboratory may be warranted.

During a formal sleep study, you will spend the night in a laboratory, hooked up to an EEG (electroencephalograph) machine with painless electrodes placed on your head. Sounds restful, doesn't it? In time, when you finally fall asleep in this weird environment, the EEG will record data regarding how long it takes you to fall asleep, how long you spend in each stage of sleep, and if you experience delta wave sleep, REM sleep, sleep myoclonus, or sleep apnea.

Less frequently, doctors may request PET scans, CT scans, or X-ray studies of various tissues or organs to determine if sleep disturbances are due to some underlying disorder.

TRIAGING YOUR TREATMENT: LESS IS MORE

Okay. You've got the doctor and you've got the test results. Now for the moment you've been waiting for: relief!

With so many possible symptoms, dozens of possible coexisting problems, and even more potential therapies, where in the world do you and your physician start the treatment process?

Unfortunately, many practitioners start (and end) with whatever limited treatments they already know, can offer themselves, or have recommended in the past. This is a red flag to go elsewhere. Wise physicians don't start with their favorite treatments, they start with each individual patient, one patient at a time.

Developing an individual treatment plan that provides real and lasting relief requires prioritizing your problems, a process known as *triage*. You and your doctor should discuss which problems to tackle first and which can wait a little longer.

As I mentioned before, if there is an emergency, go directly to the emergency room of the nearest hospital or urgent care center. If you are experiencing seizures from taking a medication, chest pain, severe dizziness, high fever, terrible pain, or other urgent problem, you need immediate help.

If the situation is not urgent—in the vast majority of fibromyalgia cases it is not—you and your physician will have to determine priorities. If tests show, for example, that you have candida overgrowth, which can eventually undermine your overall health, you may choose to treat that problem first, before focusing on your sleep disturbances, which have been occurring for quite some time and aren't getting any worse. The yeast infection can be treated with natural remedies or conventional medications, hopefully removing it from the picture. Then you can turn your attention toward solving your sleep problems. You may even find you sleep better once the yeast problem is gone.

Some symptoms can be dealt with together; other problems are best tackled one at a time. Together, you and your physician can map out a tentative game plan, with the knowledge that the list may change along the way, as various symptoms improve or worsen and test results provide more information.

LESS IS MORE

Regardless of which problem you try to solve first, the guiding principle in designing a treatment plan (for nonemergency conditions) is always to *start with the least aggressive treatments* and see if they help, before progressing to more aggressive and often riskier treatments.

In other words, start with the least you can do to achieve your goals and only do more if you have to. Although this sounds logical, there can be tremendous resistance to this approach, by both the doctor and the patient. Patients often want a quick fix, preferably in an easy-to-swallow form; and physicians generally want to do something effective as quickly as possible. Too often this combination of desires leads to premature prescriptions for medications.

But going right for conventional medicine's big guns (prescription drugs) can backfire. Try to resist the urge to ask immediately for whatever pill can help you feel better. Studies now show the fourth leading cause of death in the United States, after heart disease, cancer, and stroke, is complications due to taking medications! If that many folks are dying from taking medically prescribed drugs, think of how many more people probably get unnecessarily sick every day just from taking their medicine!

I like to start with the less aggressive treatments, including changes in lifestyle behaviors (like moving toward a plant-based diet or quitting smoking) and active self-help measures (like moderate exercise). Lifestyle changes and self-help activities (in Chapter 6) call for your active participation in the healing process. Without this, nothing your health care team offers you can really help. If you are a passive, junk-food junkie, a couch potato who smokes three packs of cigarettes a day, lives in a toxic environment, and is angry at the world, it's unlikely that conventional or CAM interventions are going to be especially effective or long lasting, no matter what pill you pop. In fact, passive interventions that don't address the underlying problems may make matters worse.

The great thing about starting with self-help therapies is it puts you in control. Your physician can help you wade through the many self-help options by providing clear information and telling what to expect as you try them. If your fibromyalgia pain is focused in your back or neck, for example, your physician might recommend a program of gentle exercises designed to improve overall flexibility and alleviate pain. He or she might tell you why exercise helps and what frequency is best. But the actual treatment—stretching three times a day, or whatever is recommended—happens only if *you* do it. Each day *you* will decide if and when you do your exercises, and only *you* will be able to determine if they are effective in reducing your pain.

Once self-help measures are well underway, the next logical step is to choose one or more of the wide variety of natural therapies available (herbs, acupuncture, bodywork, etc.), depending on your test results and ongoing symptoms. The natural therapies appropriate for fibromyalgia are described in great detail in Chapters 8 through 12.

Be patient. Many self-help and natural therapies take time to work. You probably won't see a big difference in your symptoms right away, and when you do start to see results it may be quite gradual. Try to hang in there and give these measures a chance to succeed.

EXPANDING YOUR TEAM

After you and your physician are reasonably confident in your diagnosis and you've got a good idea of what you are trying to treat, it's time to enlist the services of other health care professionals, both conventional and complementary. At the recommendation of your physician, or perhaps because of your own interest in a particular therapy, you'll be including one or more the following professionals in your team:

- **Family physicians, general practitioners, and primary-care physicians.** These doctors provide general care for adults and children. If you are seeing a specialist, you may be referred back to a primary-care physician once your symptoms are under control.

- **Nurses** may assist your physician with the management of your fibromyalgia symptoms and may be called upon to teach you about your treatments and answer many of your questions. Just as is true with many boss–secretary relationships, the person perceived to have the least power is in fact the most powerful. Doctors are not always approachable. They may not be available to return phone calls or answer questions. It behooves you to establish a trusting relationship with at least one nurse who knows your case. Ask any mother who has delivered her child in a hospital, and you'll be told that the nurses gave her more comfort and reassurance than her own doctor. Nurses are indispensable.

- **Occupational therapists (OT)** help patients with fibromyalgia conserve energy and develop adaptations necessary to continue daily life. The OT strives for a balance of work, rest, and play. To help you avoid or limit fatigue, your OT will help you devise a plan for pacing yourself, living with children, performing daily tasks at work and in and around the house, finding ways to get around and stay mobile, caring for your personal needs, and staying comfortable.

- **Pharmacists** fill your prescriptions and can explain the action of drugs and their potential side effects. They can advise you of possible drug interactions if you're taking more than one medicine, and answer your questions about over-the-counter medicines. Pharmacists may be aware of new medications that might benefit you as soon as they are available, so you can discuss them with your doctor.

- **Physical therapists (PT)** can teach you exercises to help make your muscles stronger and thus better able to support your bones and joints. They can educate you on the use of different kinds of equipment to help you improve muscle strength and can design custom exercise programs to help you meet your specific goals, such as cardiovascular health, weight loss or maintenance, or reducing stiffness. Your PT may treat symptoms with such agents as heat, cold, electrical current, and mechanical apparatus. He or she may offer massage, myofascial release, stretching, acupressure, aerobic exercise program, and adaptive equipment.

- **Physician's assistants** are trained, certified, and licensed professionals who assist physicians by taking patient histories, performing physical examinations, making diagnoses, and designing treatments. They work under the supervision of a physician.

- **Podiatrists** specialize in foot care. Many work in conjunction with chiropractors to help ensure you get the most from your shoes. The type of shoe you wear is important in terms of support. Many fibromyalgia sufferers have poor biomechanics and posture and can find relief and improvement in proper foot support.

- **Social workers** can help you find solutions to social and financial problems related to your disorder. A social worker will be especially important if you have no health insurance or if your fibromyalgia is so severe that you need disability benefits.

- **Psychiatrists** can help you deal with depression, anxiety, and other mental problems related to fibromyalgia. They are medical doctors and can prescribe medications.

- **Psychologists** can help you deal with depression, anxiety, and other mental problems but cannot prescribe medications.

- **A variety of CAM practitioners** (see Chapters 7 to 12), including acupuncturists, chiropractors, herbalists, massage therapists, dietitians, and nutritionists.

MANAGING YOUR TEAM

Although your health care team probably won't include all the professionals just listed, even adding one, two, or three more experts will improve your odds of feeling better faster, especially if everyone works together and shares information. While each practitioner will focus on his or her specialty, it's important to remember the big picture: an integrative approach to better health. *You* are the boss, the team manager, along with your comanager, your physician.

Here's how to get the most out of your team:

- Engage only those health care providers who treat you with respect. Health care professionals who do their jobs well have no reason to feel threatened by your involvement.
- Ask every provider for copies of any test results and reports, and make sure you understand what the records mean.
- Keep a daily journal on your condition, especially regarding symptoms and what helps and hurts (see Chapter 2).
- Take notes whenever a member of your health care team talks to you about your disorder. You may want to bring a small, inexpensive tape

recorder to your doctor's office and to your therapy sessions. Reviewing your notes or the tape will help you understand what you've been told and formulate questions.

- Finally, keep an open mind about your team and be flexible regarding members. You may find yourself consulting with practitioners whose specialties are unfamiliar to you. Just as we don't fully understand the underlying cause of fibromyalgia, we don't know the exact mechanism by which many natural therapies work. What we do know, however, is that for many patients, natural therapies can make a genuine difference. Hopefully, some of the CAM approaches will work for you, too.

MEDICATIONS FOR FIBROMYALGIA: WEIGHING THE RISKS, REAPING THE BENEFITS

If, after first trying self-help activities and then some of the natural therapies, some of your fibromyalgia symptoms are still not under control, you and your physician may be ready to explore conventional medications. Again, I prefer to use a less is more approach when selecting and recommending drugs, starting with the milder medications that carry the least offensive or least potentially dangerous side effects.

As I mentioned in Chapter 2, there's no free ride: *All conventional medications can have potentially negative side effects.* That's why every decision regarding medication should involve an open discussion about potential risks and possible benefits. In medicine, as in most of life, nothing is black or white, all good or all bad. There are only shades of gray and we must continuously choose among the best of all current options.

When deciding whether or not to use medications, it's essential to gather enough information to make an informed decision. This includes talking to your doctor. Whether you make the decision with the help of others or entirely on your own, you must *inform your physician* so he or she can help coordinate your care. Some medications do not mix well with one another or with other substances, like herbs or even some foods. Make sure you tell your doctor about *all* your current medications and treatments.

The following discussion of medications sometimes used in the treatment of fibromyalgia is for informational purposes only and is not intended to be a substitute for experienced medical advice from your licensed physician. With that in mind, here is a long (but far from exhaustive) list of potential medications.

GENERALLY HELPFUL
FIBROMYALGIA MEDICATIONS

There are some medicines that seem to help most fibromyalgia patients even if no underlying causes are identified. A good example of a class of drugs that tends to help patients with fibromyalgia are tricyclic antidepressants (TCAs). TCAs have been helping people with depression and other problems for 40 years or so.

To treat fibromyalgia, physicians often prescribe lower doses than normally given to alleviate depression. Experience shows that TCAs are effective in treating a number of symptoms associated with fibromyalgia. Sleep is often improved, probably because these drugs increase the amount of delta wave sleep. They also make serotonin more readily available to cells and heighten the effect of endorphins, both of which help relieve pain.

Unlike other powerful pain relievers such as morphine, TCAs are not addicting. Side effects you may experience include increased drowsiness (although 10 to 15 percent of patients actually become more energetic), dry mouth, blurred vision, constipation, low blood pressure, and heart palpitations. Many of these adverse reactions can be alleviated by lowering the dosage. Finding the right TCA and the right dosage for you is important and may take some time. The TCAs include *Sinequan (doxepin)* and *Elavil (amitriptyline)*. These can be helpful at bedtime for reducing sleep disturbances and depression and will also tend to raise the pain threshold over time.

Other medicines that generally tend to be helpful with fibromyalgia include:

> *Flexeril (cyclobenzaprine)*—primarily a muscle relaxer; affects the central nervous system and helps induce sleep. Studies show this medication loses its effect when taken regularly over long periods. Does not reduce morning stiffness.

Neurontin (gabapentin)—an anticonvulsant that helps relieve chronic pain by increasing the level of gamma-aminobutyric acid (GABA), which slows down nerve impulses. GABA also blocks the release of excitatory amino acids, which promote chronic pain.

Guaifenesin—(normally used as an expectorant) and *dextromethorphan* (normally used as a cough suppressant)—in prescription doses can be helpful in treating chronic pain in some patients. Guaifenesin works in a different manner than Neurontin, however. It thins out secretions, and in so doing, may make it easier for cells to pick up nutrients and get rid of wastes. Dextromethorphan's pain-relieving properties are thought to be related to its action on endorphin receptors.

IMPORTANT *TARGETED* MEDICATIONS TO CONSIDER FOR FIBROMYALGIA SYMPTOMS AND RELATED PROBLEMS

- *Coumadin* or *heparin* (blood thinners)—a subset of fibromyalgia patients appear to have an overactive clotting mechanism that causes the blood to thicken slightly and impairs circulation. Small doses of these medicines can thin the blood to the normal range and reduce pain. Coumadin, in the larger, more commonly prescribed doses, causes significant risk of bleeding, but in tiny doses, with periodic monitoring, carries next to no risk.

- *Lamisil (terbinafine)* or *Diflucan (fluconazole)*— for laboratory-diagnosed candida overgrowth. Do not take these if you have liver disease.

- *Nystatin*—effective in treating mucosal candida overgrowth.

- *Doxycycline, tetracycline,* or *Biaxin (clarithromycin)*—for treating fibromyalgia patients who have laboratory evidence of a chronic infection with mycoplasma, an atypical bacteria that multiplies inside, rather than outside cells.

- *Thyroid medicine*—may help sufferers of fibromyalgia with documented marginal or abnormal thyroid function. Monitor blood tests to prevent overtreatment.

- *Natural hormones*—to correct hormonal imbalances. Do not take unless tests reveal an imbalance.

- *DHEA* and/or *pregnenolone*—adrenal gland hormones that may help decrease fatigue and improve sleep. Recent studies suggest DHEA may somehow reduce "foggy" thinking. Use DHEA with great care, only when the levels are low, with medical supervision and monitoring. In men with prostate cancer and women with early gynecologic cancer, cancer may become more aggressive with higher levels of DHEA.

- *Cortisol*—adjust dosage by blood testing to prevent overtreatment.

- *Florinef (fludrocortisone acetate)*—in the morning or *DDAVP nasal spray (desmopressin acetate)* in the evening, if the blood pressure tends to be low.

INJECTABLE MEDICINES

- *Trigger point (not tender point) injections* of *lidocaine or Marcaine*—may provide temporary pain relief. A common intervention when a fibromyalgia patient has pain in a specific location, such as the lower back or neck. Usually involves three injections per visit, with visits spaced several weeks apart. Each injection contains an anesthetic, such as Marcaine. The trigger point is often sprayed with a cooling anesthetic to numb the area before injection.
- *Intramuscular injections* of B_{12}, *magnesium, B_6, Kutapressin, and other compounds*—used widely for fatigue and pain.
- *Intravenous infusions of a Meyer's cocktail* (magnesium, calcium, vitamin C, and the B vitamins)—usually given weekly for four to six weeks to improve muscle aches and fatigue.
- *Growth hormone shots*—if levels are low.

MEDICATIONS FOR PAIN AND BETTER SLEEP

A number of medications are commonly prescribed for managing fibromyalgia pain and sleep disturbances. Depending on your situation, your physician may advise you to take one of the following:

- *Ambien (zolpidem)*—a sleep medicine that tends to be less addictive than the benzodiazepines.

- *EMLA cream*—prescription topical cream that may help reduce the sensitivity of skin trigger points for pain.
- *Imitrex*—used for migraine headache pain.
- *Klonopin (klonazepam)*—a benzodiazepine used to combat muscle twitching, restless leg syndrome, and anxiety. Does nothing for pain, but it does promote restful sleep by alleviating other symptoms. The most common side effect is fatigue. It makes you sleepy! Effects decrease with time, and there is the potential for addiction after just several weeks of use.
- *Paxil (paroxetine HCl)*—a selective serotonin reuptake inhibitor (SSRI) that reduces uptake of the neurotransmitter serotonin and may reduce pain.
- *Celebrex (celecoxib) or Vioxx rufecoxib*—a new class of nonsteroidal anti-inflammatory medications that have a much lower incidence of side effects, such as gastritis or gastrointestinal bleeding.
- *Ultram (tramadol HCl)*—for moderate to severe pain. Changes how the central nervous system processes pain. Does not provide a "high," so people aren't motivated to take it other than for pain relief. Side effects may include constipation, dizziness, nausea, headaches, and vomiting.
- *Narcotic medicines*, such as the potent pain reliever morphine or other opium derivatives. Very effective at pain relief. Their use can cause

drowsiness, stupor, euphoria, sedation, or constipation, and may aggravate depression and sleep disturbances. They are highly addictive, so avoid unless absolutely necessary.

SUPPLEMENT/DRUG INTERACTIONS— RECIPES FOR DISASTER

As noted earlier, the use of complementary/alternative medicine in North America is on the rise. Dr. David Eisenberg, who surveyed 1,539 adults in 1990 and 2,055 adults in 1997, found that the use of CAM increased from 33.8 percent to 42.1 percent of the population over the seven-year period. Although this constitutes a 25 percent increase, certain slices of the CAM pie have grown even more rapidly. In particular, the use of high-dose vitamins has increased 130 percent and the use of herbal supplements has grown 380 percent between 1990 and 1997.

Almost one in five patients taking prescription medicines are also taking herbs, high-dose vitamins, or both. However, most of these individuals don't tell their physicians about their general use of CAM and supplements in particular. This means about 15 million adults in the United States are at risk for potential interactions between their medications and supplements. Some of these interactions are relatively benign, while others can be potentially life-threatening.

The number of possible interactions between supplements and medications is overwhelming. We need to be especially careful when mixing supplements or herbs with drugs that have a narrow therapeutic window*, control potentially life-threatening conditions, or are notorious for toxic interactions. These drugs or classes of drugs include:

- **Antiarrhythmics** (particularly digoxin*)
- **Antiasthmatics** (particularly theophylline*)
- **Anticoagulants** (particularly Coumadin*)
- **Anticonvulsants*** (such as Dilantin or Depakote)
- **Antidepressants** (particularly MAOIs, like Nardil and Parnate; and SSRIs, such as Celexa, Paxil, Prozac, and Zoloft)
- **Antidiabetics*** (both insulin and oral hypoglycemics)
- **Antihypertensives**
- **Hepatotoxic agents** (drugs that can cause liver damage, including Accutane, cyclosporine, Leukine, and Prograf)
- **Immunosuppressants** (cortisone, cyclosporine, methotrexate, prednisone, and others)
- **Nephrotoxic agents** (drugs that can cause kidney toxicity, including some antibiotics such as gentamicin and tobramycin; some chemotherapy drugs like cisplatin and mitomycin; cyclosporine; Prograf; and Vistide)

---

* Drugs with a "narrow therapeutic window" are ineffective at low doses and can cause dangerous side effects at high doses. Despite FDA assurances of equivalency, many doctors feel it's best to avoid generic substitutes for these medications.

> If you are taking any of the medications just list-
> ed, it is *vital* that you talk to your physician, or
> someone knowledgeable about drug and supple-
> ment interactions, *before* taking any other med-
> ication, supplement, or herbal remedy.

NONDRUG MEDICAL TREATMENTS
FOR FIBROMYALGIA

In addition to medications, conventional medicine does
have a few other ways to treat the symptoms of
fibromyalgia and related disorders. Although typically
grouped with the complementary/alternative interventions, they do offer low-risk alternatives to conventional medications. Three that I sometimes recommend
to my patients are topical capsaicin creams, ultrasound
therapy, and the use of a transcutaneous electrical
nerve stimulator (TENS). As always, please consult
with your physician before pursuing these or any other
treatments.

CAPSAICIN CREAMS

Capsaicin is an ingredient derived from hot peppers.
This used to be a prescription item but is now readily
available over the counter. Although initially irritating,
the repeated application of capsaicin cream over painful
areas does reduce chronic pain by depleting Substance P

(which is elevated in chronic pain sufferers). It's generally advisable to start with the lowest strength you can find, applied to a small area. Once you have worked through the initial irritating phase, you can apply stronger creams to larger areas.

ULTRASOUND THERAPY

Ultrasound therapy delivers high-frequency heat therapy to an injury site or area of chronic pain. The technique is generally used in the context of physical therapy to increase local circulation and decrease inflammation. It can also be an effective way to stretch and soften scar tissue and even reduce muscle spasms.

Ultrasound therapy is delivered in either a pulse or continuous mode. Physiotherapists generally use the continuous mode on patients who have chronic injuries, and the pulse mode on those with acute injuries. In continuous mode, the patient may feel a warming sensation at the treatment site. The practitioner applies a special gel (which enhances transmission of the ultrasound waves) to the individual's skin before commencing therapy. The ultrasound waves generate vibrations and heat deep in the tissues, which can improve circulation and help break down scar tissue.

TRANSCUTANEOUS ELECTRICAL NERVE STIMULATOR (TENS)

The transcutaneous electrical nerve stimulator is a small, battery-operated device that produces various frequencies and voltages of mild electrical stimulation; it is used frequently in the management of chronic pain. By applying the electrodes to painful areas, the electric current acts upon the nerves, blocking the pain. TENS units are also though to stimulate the production of endorphins. Patients can be taught by a physician or therapist to administer this treatment themselves.

4

Eat Better, Feel Better

Each day you have a new opportunity to reinvent yourself. With every breath you take, every meal you eat, every drink you swallow, you are literally building a new you. Day in and day out, you lose millions of cells from your body. And simultaneously, you take in new building materials to reconstruct yourself—new atoms, molecules, and compounds from the air you breathe and from the food and drink you consume.

Each day, as you recreate yourself, remember this: *You are an important person worthy of the best building materials!* Good nutrition is not just some nice little "extra" in life, like good table manners or nice penmanship. Good nutrition is essential to creating the healthy life you want and deserve. Every day, from this day forward, your future is in your own hands.

Eating a healthy, well-balanced diet of fresh, whole foods is the key to good health and optimal healing. Most nutritionists, registered dietitians, and other health care providers favor a whole-foods diet that emphasizes plant-based foods—vegetables, fruits, legumes (beans), and whole grains. Other foods included in a whole-foods plan are reasonable amounts of fish, poultry, and low-fat dairy products. What this diet limits is the intake of red meats, high-fat foods, sugar, sodium, and processed foods.

Eating healthy food can ease your physical discomfort, strengthen your immune system, and help you cope with whatever life throws your way. When faced with a challenge like fibromyalgia, this can mean less pain, fewer symptoms, better stamina, and an improved sense of well-being.

Too many people, however, take the "Band-Aid" approach to nutrition. Given our busy lives, it's easy to understand why lots of folks look for quick fixes in the form of convenience foods bolstered by nutritional supplements and the occasional healthy meal.

The trouble is, quick fixes just don't work. If your breakfast, lunch, and dinner consist mostly of fast foods or processed foods like frozen entrees or conveniently pack-aged soups and salads, you aren't going to combat fatigue or promote healing simply by eating an occasional cup of yogurt or popping a vitamin pill. When it comes to long-term health, there is absolutely no substitute for the positive impact of a diet composed of whole, nutrient-rich, real foods. Nutritional supplements can help make up for the "rough spots," but they won't erase the nutritional damage created by a diet of junk foods high in salt, fat, and sugar, or processed foods loaded with refined white flour, partially hydrogenated oils, preservatives, artificial flavorings, and dyes. The bottom line is you must *eat better to feel better.*

WHAT'S TO EAT?

No single magic menu fits every person at every stage of life. We each have a unique genetic and biochemical make-up, and each of us thrives on very different diets depending on our different circumstances. For example, adults with high blood triglycerides and low HDL levels may do better on a reduced-carbohydrate diet. Many children thrive on lots of complex carbohydrates and moderate protein. Some people feel their best when they follow Ayurvedic dietary guidelines; others prefer the traditional Chinese medical diet (both of these are discussed later in this book).

The basic principles of good eating are still the subject of much debate. It seems like every time we turn around, yet another "expert" is recommending some newfangled way to eat right.

Lately there's been a lot of talk about working toward "optimal ratios" and percentages. We've been told, for example, to be sure that no more than 30 percent of our calories come from fats. We hear that we should consume about 30 grams of fiber daily. We've gotten so caught up in ratios and statistics that we've lost sight of the primary focus of optimal nutrition: the actual *foods* we eat. When you choose a diet based only on grams of this or percentages of that, you miss the point of good nutrition. A meal of butter, soda, and beef jerky can give you exactly the "right" ratios of fats, carbohydrates, and protein, but where does it leave you nutritionally?

Rather than micro-managing the numbers, it makes more sense to chose *whole, unprocessed, living foods*—the kind of foods humans thrived on for thousands of years before we invented food processing factories, Wonder Bread, and solar-powered calculators to figure the nutrient ratios. Instead of crunching the numbers, we ought to be crunching real foods:

- Vegetables
- Fruits
- Whole grains
- Legumes (beans)

The most striking thing about this list of "power foods" is that they all come from plants. That doesn't mean you need to go entirely vegetarian (although it certainly wouldn't hurt). Contrary to popular myth, people who choose vegan diets (eliminating all animal products, including meat, fish, chicken, eggs, and dairy) can get all the protein and other nutrients they need from vegetables, fruits, grains, beans, nuts, and seeds.

But whatever you choose, the secret to smart eating is to select the freshest, most nutrient-rich foods available. The standard American diet is currently dominated by animal foods like meat and eggs. As a result, we consume too much protein and fat, too little fiber, and not enough of the vital nutrients. The fastest, simplest way to improve your diet is to *gradually* increase your intake of plant-based foods while decreasing the amount and frequency of animal foods.

Plant foods are truly the nutrition superstars. Plant-based diets are brimming with key nutrients—far more than you get from eating mostly animal foods. Whole grains, fruits, vegetables, and legumes provide vitamin A, vitamin C, antioxidants, all sorts of important minerals, and a fascinating family of compounds called *phytonutrients*.

Phytonutrients (sometimes called phytochemicals; *phyto* is the Latin word for plant) are health-supporting substances that occur naturally in plants and give them color, flavor, and natural disease resistance. You could live without phytonutrients, but you wouldn't live well for long. Scientists have already identified several thousand phytonutrients, and new ones are being discovered all the time. Hundreds of studies support the conclusion that these plant compounds with impossible-to-pronounce Latin names may be our nutritional guardian angels, offering natural protection against many kinds of cancer and reducing the risk of heart disease and even memory loss. Each phytonutrient has its own health-promoting action, but they all complement one another in boosting the body's defense system, enhancing the absorption of nutrients, and eliminating cellular waste.

Fresh fruits, vegetables, whole grains, and legumes deliver an incredible number of phytonutrients—including 800 bioflavonoids, 450 carotenoids, and 150 anthocyanins. You may have already heard about some of them:

- *Lycopene* is a member of the carotene family found in cooked tomatoes; it gives tomatoes their red color and is associated with a lower incidence of cancers of the breast, lung, digestive tract, and prostate, as well as reduced risk of memory loss.

- *Sulfurophane* is a phytochemical found in broccoli, cauliflower, and other cruciferous vegetables; it boosts key cancer-fighting enzymes that remove carcinogens from cells before they can do damage.
- *Resveratrol* is a powerful phytochemical found in grapes and red wine; it helps control oxidative damage.
- *Zeaxanthin* is a color molecule found in green leafy vegetables; it helps filter out damaging ultraviolet light and protects your eyes.
- *Saponins* are found in beans and legumes; they are thought to prevent cancer cells from multiplying.
- *Genistein* is found in soybean products; it starves tumors by interfering with the formation of capillaries that carry nutrients to them.

In addition to these phytonutrients, most plants are full of fiber. Fiber comes in two major types. Soluble fiber absorbs water and helps lower cholesterol levels (think of Metamucil or oatmeal). Insoluble fiber (vegetables and bran) does not absorb water and helps prevent colon cancer, heart disease, diabetes, diverticulosis, and constipation. Aim to make fiber-rich foods an important component of your diet. Experts recommend 25 to 35 grams of fiber per day. Most people get less than half of that.

RDAs and DRIs

The Recommended Dietary Allowances (RDAs) were developed to guide meal planning for institutions like hospitals and schools. The nutrition guidelines were intended to help the public avoid dietary deficiency diseases such as scurvy, pellagra, and beriberi. When was the last time you heard of anyone having a deficiency disease? Today most people are not worried about beriberi; they're looking for ways to achieve optimal health and healing. The RDAs, though a useful starting point, are considered largely inadequate today.

In the mid-1990s the National Academy of Sciences helped shift the thinking on nutrition recommendations by issuing Dietary Reference Intakes (DRIs), revised guidelines that focused on optimal health and bumped up the recommended ranges for many key nutrients. The DRIs tell us, for example, not only how much vitamin C we need to prevent scurvy, but also how much we need for the best antioxidant protection in order to maintain good health under conditions of physical and emotional stress. The DRIs also give us information on safe and adequate levels and suggest an upper limit for each nutrient.

Basic Dietary Guidelines

These are the food recommendations established jointly by the U.S. Departments of Agriculture (USDA) and Health and Human Services.

Breads, Cereals, Rice, and Pasta—Try to get 6 to 11 servings from this group daily. These foods supply complex carbohydrates, fiber, and minerals. One serving equals 1 slice of bread; ½ cup cooked cereal, rice, or pasta; ½ small bagel or muffin; or 1 ounce dry cereal. For maximum fiber, use whole grain products.

Fruits—Reach for 2 to 4 servings daily. Fruits provide vitamins A and C, potassium, and fiber. One serving equals 1 medium apple, banana, orange, or peach; ½ cup chopped, cooked, or canned fruit; or ¾ cup juice.

Vegetables—Go for 3 to 5 servings daily. Vegetables, especially the deep-yellow and deep-green varieties, are packed with vitamins, minerals, and fiber. One serving equals 1 cup raw leafy greens, ½ cup cooked vegetables, or ¾ cup juice.

Meat, Poultry, Fish, Dried Beans, Eggs, and Nuts—Get 2 to 3 servings daily from this group. These foods are sources of protein, B vitamins, iron, and zinc. One serving equals 2 to 3 ounces of cooked lean meat, poultry, or fish (about the size of a deck of cards); 1 egg; or ½ cup cooked beans. To keep fat intake low, choose legumes, lean meats and fish, and skinless poultry breast meat.

Milk, Yogurt, and Cheese—Aim for 2 to 3 servings from this group. Dairy products are a source of protein, vitamins, and minerals—especially calcium and some B vitamins. One serving equals 1 cup (8 ounces) of milk or yogurt; 1 ½ ounces of a natural cheese, such as cheddar or Swiss; or 2 ounces of processed cheese, such as American. Use fat-free or reduced-fat products to keep your fat intake low.

Fats, Oils, and Sweets—Limit intake. This group includes butter, margarine, oils, candy, soda, cakes, cookies, and similar foods. One serving equals 1 teaspoon of butter, margarine, or oil.

MUNCHING THE MACRONUTRIENTS: PROTEINS, CARBOHYDRATES, AND FATS

You get your energy from eating macronutrients. "Macro" simply means large. Relatively speaking, your diet consists of large amounts of proteins, carbohydrates, and fats (which are measured in grams), compared to vitamins, minerals, and other micronutrients (which are measured in milligrams, one thousandth of a gram).

Calories simply measure how much energy is contained in food. Think of the number of calories you eat each day as an amount of money available to spend. There is no one perfect way to spend that money, just like there is no one perfect diet. But you do not want to blow your budget on "trinkets" and have nothing of lasting value to show for it in return. Similarly, try to spend your calories wisely by choosing a nutrient-dense diet.

To consume fewer calories without losing important nutrients, build your diet around nutrient-rich, unprocessed whole grains, fruits, and vegetables. Shun the nutrient-poor foods, such as soda, chips, candy, and cake. Collard greens, for example, have only 40 calories per half cup and provide 3.6 grams (g) of protein, 400 milligrams (mg) of potassium, 178 mg of calcium, 1 mg iron, and 6,500 International Units (IU) of vitamin A. Compare that with a 40-calorie serving of coffee cake (just one bite!), which provides less than 1 g of protein, 1 g of fat, no calcium, 10 mg of potassium, and 2 IU of vitamin A.

This doesn't mean you can never eat coffee cake or other nutrient-deficient foods. Just be aware of how you are spending your calories—your nutritional cash—so that by the end of the day, you've invested wisely.

PROTEINS

In a plant-based diet *at least three-quarters* of the food on your plate should come from grains, fruits, and vegetables. Most Americans were raised on a diet that is just the opposite, with large servings of meat, fish, and chicken, and smaller portions of "side dishes." Building your diet around animal foods is counter-productive, because when you fill up on proteins, you have less room for the vitamin-rich foods that are your best sources of phytonutrients, antioxidants, and fiber. If you do eat animal protein, limit yourself to 2 or 3 ounces per meal—a serving size no larger than a deck of playing cards.

Rest assured, a plant-based diet is *not* a low-protein diet. The RDA for adults age 50 and under is 0.8 grams of protein per kilogram of body weight, or about .36 grams for every pound you weigh. This means a woman who weighs 130 pounds (59 kg) needs only 47.2 g of protein per day to meet the RDA.

Even vegetarians can get enough protein. Not long ago, vegetarians were advised to follow some pretty strict guidelines. That's because some nutritionists believed that certain amino acids had to be eaten together (at the same meal) in specific combinations in order to provide "complete" proteins. The theory was that plant proteins were "incomplete" and needed to be combined with the "complementary proteins" found in beans, nuts, or grains to make a truly nutritious vegetarian meal. We now know this is untrue. Your body can use the amino acids consumed at breakfast and combine these with different amino acids consumed at lunch or dinner to make all the proteins it needs during the day.

When you opt for a plant-based diet, you can still get plenty of protein by replacing the animal protein with vegetable protein found in legumes (for example, pinto beans, black beans, split peas, or black-eyed peas), grains, soy products, meat analogs (soy hot dogs or veggie burgers), nuts, and seeds. Soy protein has been shown to lower cholesterol and may prevent cancer. If these foods are new to you, introduce them gradually, but steadily, into your diet. Be daring. Try split pea soup and a veggie burger for dinner tonight!

CARBOHYDRATES

Nutritionists continue to argue over what is the optimal amount of carbohydrates in the diet, but most experts agree that most of your calories should come from carbohydrates. The body uses carbohydrates (or starches, as grandma used to call them) to make blood sugar, which provides the fuel used by the brain and the muscles, including the heart.

Because they break down into sugar slowly, complex carbohydrates—like corn, potatoes, whole wheat bread, oats, and legumes—are far better for you than the simple carbohydrates found in sugary cereals, pies, cakes, cookies, and other processed foods made from white sugar and/or white flour. Whole grain breads and cereals are the best sources of complex carbohydrates because they also provide iron, B vitamins, and fiber—contributing nicely to the 25 to 35 g of fiber needed daily.

The USDA Food Guide Pyramid recommends 6 to 11 servings of grains per day. That sounds like an awful lot until you realize that one serving equals one slice of bread or one ounce of dry cereal. A big bagel represents four servings of grains! For best nutrition, choose one made with whole wheat flour and, for goodness sake, don't ruin it with a thick layer of butter or cream cheese. If you want a tasty topping, choose a fruit spread or some hummus (a Middle Eastern dish made from mashed chickpeas, sesame seed paste, and other healthy ingredients).

Make sure that at least half the grains you eat are whole grains, rather than white flour. When whole wheat flour is milled into white flour, 25 nutrients are lost, and only five nutrients are added back (to give you so-called "enriched" flour). Some good choices include whole wheat pasta, whole wheat bread, oatmeal, and brown rice. Try a different grain each week. Whole grains like quinoa and millet are great-tasting and easy to cook.

In addition to whole grains, fruits and vegetables are also excellent sources of complex carbohydrates. Scientific research continually supports the fact that diets high in nutrient-rich fruits and vegetables promote optimal health. Ever see a study saying broccoli is bad for you? One study showed that people who consumed lots of fruits and vegetables had the lowest heart attack rates and cut their risk of developing certain cancers by half.

The USDA Food Guide Pyramid recommends getting five to nine servings of fruits and vegetables per day. Yes, five to nine servings. "Five a day" is a great slogan, but research shows five is really not enough. Eating nine servings may seem difficult, but if you start your day with a glass of juice and some fruit on your cereal, you've already packed in two servings right there with breakfast. Help yourself to a vegetable at lunch and two more at dinner. Snack on fresh fruit or cut-up raw vegetables. You'll find you've reached your goal in no time. An easy way to get enough vegetables is to double your portion size. If you eat a full cup of broccoli at dinner you've eaten two servings instead of just one!

Sugar

Although the complex carbohydrates found in whole grains and vegetables are good for you, the simple carbohydrates (a.k.a. sugar) should be avoided. That means no sugary sodas, juices, candies, or desserts. Some studies show sugar can impair the action of white blood cells, rendering your immune system less effective. Since many people with fibromyalgia get frequent infections, you don't want to eat in ways that could further compromise your immune system. Furthermore, for those fibromyalgia patients with evidence of candida overgrowth syndrome (COS), a diet high in sugar can facilitate candida/yeast overgrowth.

You've heard it before: sugar provides "empty calories." Most of the sugar Americans consume does not come from the sugar bowl on the table, but is hidden in our foods. Check the labels of your favorite pizza sauce, ketchup, cereal, cookies, and frozen desserts for hidden sugar in the form of sucrose, glucose, dextrose, fructose, maltose, lactose, corn syrup, or honey (usually listed in the first four ingredients on the label). By any name, it is still sugar. It is best to avoid it altogether. That said, having an *occasional* sweet with a meal is not the end of the world, because there is less of a sugar effect when the sweet is diluted by other dietary elements.

Sugar Substitutes

Limiting sugar does not mean you should move over to the artificial sugar substitutes. Aspartame, sold as Nutrasweet or Equal, is a common trigger for headaches. People with fibromyalgia often have weak immune systems and neurological problems, and aspartame could potentially aggravate these conditions. While some people can consume aspartame without apparent negative effects, many find it does cause problems, especially when consumed in soft drinks or in between-meal snacks when no other food is being ingested. Since no one *needs* sugar substitutes, it is probably best to avoid them altogether.

Here is a sensible approach. If a food really needs some sweetening, a tiny bit of sugar is OK, especially as part of a meal. For example, if a touch of brown sugar will induce you to eat a big bowl of organic oatmeal, go for it. Better yet, add natural sweeteners, like fruit juice or fresh fruits. You could also try an herbal alternative called stevia, a sweet-tasting plant that makes a nice sugar substitute. Try it on your morning oatmeal.

FATS: THE GOOD, THE BAD, AND THE UGLY

Health authorities are still arguing over the best level of fat in the diet, but most of us would do well to cut back on our fats. Dean Ornish, a physician at Stanford University, showed that heart disease could be reversed by eating a diet in which only 10 percent of calories came from fat, as part of an overall program that included stress reduction, exercise, and meditation. On the other hand, some high-fat foods not generally included in the Ornish diet are associated with health-protective effects. A large study done at Loma Linda University showed that nut consumption is associated with protection against heart disease and with decreased risk of death from all causes.

Not all fats are the same. While experts debate the merits and amounts of dietary fat, everyone seems to agree that saturated fat should be limited. Saturated fat is found in red meat and in solid shortening. Hydrogenated oil is a type of saturated fat made when liquid oil is chemically treated with hydrogen to make it solid at room temperature. Hydrogenated fats are used in margarine and in processed foods like crackers, cookies, and chips. Hydrogenation creates trans fatty acids, which increase the risk of cancer and heart disease. Hydrogenated oils also tend to increase inflammatory substances in the body and cause cell membrane dysfunction—the last thing fibromyalgia patients need.

Eliminate as many saturated fats and hydrogenated oils from your diet as you possibly can. An excellent start is to reduce animal foods as well as processed foods like potato chips and commercially made cookies.

Polyunsaturated fats are found in soy oil, corn oil, and other vegetable oils. These can be used in moderation, but it's still wise to avoid deep-fried foods. Frying tends to damage the unstable polyunsaturated fats and increases their carcinogenic quality. Diets very high in polyunsaturated fats may be associated with certain cancers. Moderation is the key.

When it comes to fats, monounsaturated fats (found in olives, olive oil, and canola oil); occasional servings of certain high-fat foods (such as nuts, nut butters, full-fat soy foods, and avocados); and omega-3 fatty acids (found in fatty fish such as salmon, flaxseed, and fish oil capsules) may be the best bets overall. Let's take a closer look at these omega-3 fatty acids.

Essential Fatty Acids

Some fats are protective, and two in particular are essential to health—linolenic acid (omega-6) and alpha-linolenic acid (omega-3). These essential fatty acids make up the outer coating of every cell in your body. They're also needed for the proper development and functioning of the brain and nervous system and for the production of hormone-like substances called eico-sanoids (thromboxanes, leukotrienes, and prostaglandins). These chemicals regulate numerous body functions including blood pressure, the immune system, and inflammatory responses.

It is important to remember that omega-6 and omega-3 fatty acids are not interchangeable; you must consume both. These two families of essential fatty acids compete in the body, so eating too many omega-6 fatty acids may compromise omega-3 status. Research suggests that balanced levels of essential fatty acids may play a critical role in the development or prevention of chronic diseases including coronary artery disease, hypertension, Type II diabetes, arthritis and other immune/inflammatory disorders, and cancer.

Many foods contain omega-6 essential fatty acids: seeds, nuts, grains, and legumes like soy. Omega-3 fatty acids are not as plentiful in our food supply. The primary source for most Americans is fish.

Just the Flax, Ma'am

Flax and flaxseed oil are excellent sources of omega-3 fatty acids. Seven grams of flaxseed oil is equivalent to 1 g of fish oil. Try a daily dose of 3 heaping tablespoons (approximately 25 to 30 g) of ground flaxseed or 1 to 3 teaspoons of cold-pressed flaxseed oil. Flaxseed oil is highly unsaturated and is easily damaged when exposed to light, heat, or air. It is therefore generally packaged in black plastic or dark brown glass bottles to protect it from light. The oil must be refrigerated and stays fresh for up to eight weeks after it's opened.

You don't benefit from the omega-3 in whole flaxseed unless you grind the seeds in a coffee grinder or food processor. The whole seeds are protected by a hard outer coat and generally pass through the body undigested.

If you use your grinder for coffee, first grind a couple of tablespoons of white rice to get rid of the coffee taste. Toss the rice, wipe out the grinder, then grind your flaxseed. Ground flaxseed can be sprinkled on salad or cereal. (The soluble fiber in the seeds absorbs liquid and thickens the cereal if it sits.) Freeze any ground flax you don't plan to use in the next few days.

Recent studies show that the essential fatty acids in flax can positively affect our immune response, which may help in the management of autoimmune diseases. By changing the fats found in cell membranes, the essential fatty acids in flax lower the production of arachidonic acid, a substance used by the body to make the chemicals that cause inflammation, such as certain types of prostaglandins and cytokines. Therefore, adding flax to the diet may help reduce symptoms of fibromyalgia, as well as those common to lupus, rheumatoid arthritis, psoriasis, ulcerative colitis, multiple sclerosis, and other autoimmune diseases.

Soy generally gets all the press for being a phyto-estrogen, a natural plant estrogen that can paradoxically both block or stimulate the actions of estrogen in the body, depending on whether there is too much or too little circulating estrogen. Yet flaxseed provides potent phytoestrogens called lignans. Populations who consume high amounts of lignans as part of a high-fiber diet tend to have fewer cases of hormone-dependent cancers such as breast and ovarian cancer.

Flax Cooking Tips

Here are some cooking tips to help you boost your flax intake:

- Try using ground flaxseed to replace eggs in your baking. One tablespoon of ground flax mixed with 3 tablespoons of liquid replaces one egg. Mix ground flaxseed and water in a small bowl and let it sit for a minute or two. Then add it to your recipe as you would an egg.
- Substitute ground flaxseed for the oil or shortening called for in a recipe. If a recipe calls for ⅓ cup of oil, use 1 cup of ground flaxseed. Substitute at a 3:1 ratio.
- If you're currently supplementing your diet with fish oil to get your essential fatty acids, try flaxseed or flax oil. Other sources include borage oil, evening primrose oil, and a green called purslane.

MAXIMIZING YOUR MICRONUTRIENTS: VITAMINS AND MINERALS

In the next chapter, we'll go into great detail about which vitamins, minerals, and herbs can supercharge your diet and help ease your fibromyalgia symptoms, but here's some news you can use right now: Regardless of your health or diet, you should take a multivitamin and mineral supplement every day.

Given the currently depleted condition of our farm soils and the rush and stress of modern life, no one eats a perfect diet. Daily supplementation can serve as your nutritional "insurance policy." Skeptics argue that eating a well-balanced diet provides all the nutrition you need and that taking supplements just makes "expensive urine." While everyone should strive for a well-balanced diet (and not take supplements as a substitute for eating healthy food), research shows that we would have to eat huge amounts of some foods to get enough vitamins and other nutrients to prevent disease and optimize health. It's certainly possible to get carried away and spend too much money on supplements, but a good multivitamin is an excellent investment in your overall health.

Here are the basic micronutrients we all need every day. If you have problems with digestion, take your vitamins and minerals in a powder, liquid, or chewable form instead of in capsules or tablets.

B VITAMINS

The B vitamins help us convert the food we eat into energy. They also are important to the proper functioning of the chemicals in the brain. B vitamins are used to make the "feel good" neurotransmitter serotonin. Some cases of depression have been linked to deficiencies of these critical nutrients. Be sure your multivitamin has plenty of the B vitamins. Your doctor may even suggest that you take a separate high-potency B vitamin supplement. If you have a great deal of difficulty absorbing nutrients, intravenous B vitamin therapy can sometimes be helpful. One way of figuring out if you are absorbing your B vitamins is to check the color of your urine. If your urine doesn't turn neon yellow or fluorescent orange after taking B vitamins, you may have an absorption problem.

Vitamin B₁—Also known as thiamin, this nutrient is necessary for balanced hormone levels and the metabolism of carbohydrates, fats, and proteins. B₁ helps protect your central nervous system against depression and cognitive decline. It also helps prevent the accumulation of fatty deposits in the arteries. Signs of mild B₁ deficiencies may take the form of fatigue, moodiness, skin problems, and loss of appetite. Food sources: milk, peas, legumes, soybeans, and peanuts.

Vitamin B₂—Also called riboflavin, this nutrient aids in the metabolism of carbohydrates, fats, and proteins. It helps every cell in the body use oxygen more efficiently and is also important for healthy skin and mucous membranes, good eye function, balanced hormone levels, and a healthy nervous system. It is also helpful in alleviating chronic pain. The signs of mild B₂ deficiency are wide-ranging and include cracks at the corners of the mouth, sensitivity to light, and skin rashes. Food sources: enriched grain products, some dairy products, eggs, almonds, and dark-green vegetables such as broccoli.

Vitamin B₃—commonly known as niacin, this nutrient aids digestion by helping to release energy from food. It is also involved in building red blood cells, synthesizing hormones that help you cope with stress, and promoting proper nervous system functions. When used in megadoses, niacin becomes a drug and has gotten lots of press for its cholesterol-lowering abilities. High doses have, on occasion, been associated with liver inflammation. Symptoms of mild B$_3$ deficiencies may include indigestion, appetite loss, headaches, and anxiety. Food sources: lean meats, poultry, fish, nuts and nut butters, and enriched flour.

Folate—Also commonly called folic acid or folacin, this nutrient is critical for the growth and repair of cells. It helps lower artery-clogging homocysteine levels in the blood, thereby helping to protect against heart disease. It plays a role in preventing or easing depression and in alleviating chronic pain. It can help relieve the symptoms of premenstrual syndrome (PMS) and menopause, helps protect against cervical cancer, colon cancer, heart disease, and Alzheimer's, and with pregnancy, reduces the risk of developing neural tube birth defects (like spina bifida). Food sources: avocados, asparagus, broccoli, Brussels sprouts, beans, beets, celery, corn, eggs, fish, green leafy vegetables, nuts, seeds, oatmeal, peas, orange juice, fortified cereals, and wheat germ.

Vitamin B$_5$—Also known as pantothenic acid, this nutrient is essential for food metabolism. It also aids in synthesizing hormones and encouraging normal growth and development. By supporting normal functioning of the adrenal glands, it plays a key role in the production of hormones that combat stress and ease fatigue disorders. Deficiencies of vitamin B$_5$ are extremely rare because it's readily available in so many foods, including eggs, brown rice, salmon, beans, nuts, lentils, peas, and sweet potatoes.

Vitamin B$_6$—Also known as pyridoxine, this nutrient supports the metabolism of protein and aids in the transmission of nerve impulses by supporting the production of neurotransmitters. Vitamin B$_6$ is also necessary for a healthy immune system. Because it reduces blood levels of the amino acid homocysteine, it reduces the harmful effects of cholesterol and thus helps prevent heart disease and hardening of the arteries. When prescribed in megadoses as a drug, vitamin B$_6$ may alleviate carpal tunnel syndrome and PMS. High doses, on occasion, can actually cause nerve inflammation. Signs of mild B$_6$ deficiency may include acne, insomnia, and fatigue. Food sources: whole grains, lean meats, poultry, fish, corn, nuts, potatoes, prune juice, bananas, and avocados.

Vitamin B$_{12}$—Also known as cobalamin, this nutrient is essential in metabolizing food and synthesizing red blood cells. It is sometimes called the "energy vitamin" because deficiencies (which are common in older adults and in those with digestive problems) can result in profound fatigue and depression. It also plays a critical role in producing RNA, DNA, and myelin, the protective layer over nerve endings. Symptoms of mild B$_{12}$ deficiency include weakness, fatigue, weight loss, and tingling in the arms and legs; severe deficiencies result in pernicious anemia and cognitive decline. Food sources: fish, eggs, and dairy products. Injections may be given in the case of severe deficiency.

Biotin—This nutrient works in conjunction with the other B vitamins to aid digestion by metabolizing carbohydrates, fats, and proteins. It's also key to maintaining healthy skin, hair, and nails. Signs of biotin deficiency are diverse and include hair loss, nausea, and fatigue. Food sources: cheese, salmon, sunflower seeds, nuts, broccoli, and sweet potatoes.

ANTIOXIDANT NUTRIENTS

Antioxidant nutrients include vitamin C, vitamin E, selenium, and the phytonutrients (bioflavonoids, carotenoids, and proanthocyanidins) found in fruits and vegetables. Simply speaking, raising your intake of antioxidants helps your immune system, slows down the aging process, and lowers your risk for heart disease, stroke, and cancer.

Antioxidants inhibit the chemical process known as oxidation by neutralizing the free radicals that cause oxidation. Free radicals are the unstable, highly reactive, and potentially harmful molecules formed in the body by exposure to sunlight, cigarette smoke, and environmental pollutants. Without intervention, free radicals wreak damage on the cellular level by degrading the nearest fat, protein, carbohydrate, RNA, or DNA molecule. The result is cellular decay, which hastens the aging process, damages DNA (and results in the kind of mutations that lead to cancer), and compromises the immune system (heightening your susceptibility to disease). Diseases such as arteriosclerosis, cancer, inflammatory joint disease, asthma, diabetes, senility, and diseases of the eye have all been linked to free radical damage. For example, it's thought that free radicals oxidize the LDL ("bad") cholesterol in the blood, allowing it to damage arterial walls, which leads to the blood clots and plaque formation associated with heart disease.

Vitamin C

In addition to its antioxidant benefits, vitamin C promotes and maintains healthy connective tissue (healthy collagen is critical to the maintenance of healthy joints), helps heal wounds and bruises, and stimulates the immune system to help keep disease and infection at bay.

A great deal of attention and controversy has been focused on vitamin C, thanks to the late Linus Pauling, a Nobel laureate and an outspoken advocate of megadoses of vitamin C to treat cancer and other disorders. While Pauling did stimulate important discussion, his crusade to promote high doses of vitamin C may have led him to lose sight of the importance of balance. Several studies actually document a "pro-oxidant" effect from doses of vitamin C greater than 250 mg per day. In other words, at that dosage, the vitamin can increase damage to DNA and other important cellular structures. As vitamin C neutralizes the unstable free radicals, it in turn becomes an unstable substance that needs to be neutralized.

Before you throw away your vitamin C, keep in mind that these studies were looking at vitamin C *in isolation*. Similar results have been observed with high doses of most antioxidants in isolation. However, when you look at high doses *in combination,* the opposite is true. We now know that antioxidants work best in combination, where there is antioxidant balance and not an excess of any one ingredient. By having a balanced, synergistic pool of several different types of antioxidants, it's possible to repair and recycle the damaged antioxidants back to their beneficial form.

Multivitamins generally provide vitamin C at or near the RDA of 60 mg (a level that will prevent scurvy, a deficiency disease), but there is a wealth of research that indicates this is not the optimal amount to promote health. People who smoke have lower levels of vitamin C and higher levels of free radicals, so they need extra vitamin C. For the general population, research suggests that a reasonable daily dose for preventive purposes might range from 250 mg to 1,000 mg daily in the form of a multivitamin which has a balance of antioxidants. While much higher doses of vitamin C may be used short-term for specific therapeutic interventions, chronic use of megadoses may cause problems in some people, including diarrhea and kidney stones. The body eliminates vitamin C in 12 hours. For that reason, if you're going to take a megadose of vitamin C, divide it into three smaller doses and take one with each meal. That way you'll experience the benefits of this important antioxidant around the clock.

Here are some more tips about taking vitamin C:

- Chewable vitamin C is not recommended because the acid content could possibly erode tooth enamel.
- Bioflavonoids, a type of phytonutrient found naturally in lemons and red peppers, enhance the

absorption of vitamin C when present at a level equal to or greater than the level of the vitamin C in the supplement. Unfortunately, most vitamin C supplements with bioflavonoids only add a token amount of bioflavonoids, which doesn't do much.

- Vitamin C is a diuretic, so drink plenty of fluids.
- Large amounts of vitamin C can cause diarrhea. If you develop diarrhea, decrease your daily intake.

You may have read about "rebound scurvy," a condition alleged to occur when you suddenly stop taking high doses of vitamin C. It was thought you might develop symptoms of scurvy (the vitamin C deficiency disease) because your body had become accustomed to large amounts of vitamin C. This myth has been passed along both in the scientific literature and in the popular press with little evidence to back it up.

Vitamin E

Vitamin E is an essential antioxidant that plays a major role in cardiovascular health. In the Nurses' Study at Harvard University (a long-term study involving more than eighty-seven thousand nurses begun in 1976 to look at risk factors for cancer and heart disease), women who took a daily vitamin E supplement of at least 100 IU were 34 percent less likely to have a heart attack than those who took no supplement. In the Cambridge Heart Antioxidant Study (CHAOS), an investigation involving over two thousand patients with known heart disease, vitamin E reduced nonfatal heart attack risk by 77 percent.

In 1995, the *American Journal of Clinical Nutrition* reported that scientists at the University of Naples had determined that vitamin E lowers triglyceride levels and the ratio of LDL ("bad") to HDL ("good") cholesterol, which could prevent heart disease. It also keeps arteries and veins elastic and supple, thereby preventing or easing varicose veins.

Vitamin E also helps boost your immune system. The nutrient helps counteract the natural decline in immune function associated with age by improving the function of T-cells, the blood cells that kill bacteria and viruses. A related benefit is its role in preventing or delaying the onset of cataracts, diabetes, and the cognitive degeneration associated with aging.

We don't yet know the optimal level of vitamin E on a long-term basis. Evidence suggests that the best health effects of antioxidants and other protective nutrients come from the food we eat. Try to get an adequate supply of vitamin E from food sources such as nuts and nut butters, and from vegetable oils, especially sunflower and wheat germ oil.

A few studies have suggested that people with fibromyalgia may be low in vitamin E. Since vitamin E is a powerful antioxidant that provides immune-boosting protection from free radicals, and because it is difficult to get more than about 25 IU of vitamin E from your daily diet, take a separate supplement of about 200 to 400 IU per day.

Carotenoids

The carotenoids, also referred to as carotenes, are a class of the phytonutrients discussed earlier. These are the pigment (color) molecules found in yellow-orange, red, and green vegetables, and in fruits. The term covers a family of powerful antioxidants that include beta-carotene, lycopene, and lutein. Women with higher levels of carotenoids in the blood have a lower risk for heart disease and cancer. A study of nearly seven hundred elderly nuns at the University of Kentucky found that participants with higher blood levels of lycopene functioned better overall. Who would have thought that tomato sauce could help you stay healthy as you age?

Of all the carotenes, beta-carotene is the best understood by nutritionists and the medical community. Beta-carotene is converted by the body into vitamin A. Preformed vitamin A, found in many supplements or animal products such as liver, can build up and cause liver damage. Beta-carotene does not have these toxic effects.

Beta-carotene enhances the immune system and is thought to have powerful cancer-fighting abilities. Still, studies looking into the benefits of beta-carotene have produced conflicting results. One highly publicized study found a slightly higher lung cancer rate in participants who were beta-carotene supplement users. Since carotenes are a family of nutrients, it could be that taking just beta-carotene crowds out the other members of the carotene family. For that reason, and because of the known synergy among antioxidants, I generally do not recommend taking beta-carotene supplements—or any other antioxidant or nutrient—in large doses in isolation. Having some in your multivitamin is fine, but don't take it as a single supplement. A safe and easy way to boost your beta-carotene—and get a lot of other important nutrients as well—is to drink a glass of carrot juice daily.

Proanthocyanidins

Proanthocyanidins, another type of phytonutrient, are highly potent antioxidants found in the pigment molecules of berries, pine bark, bilberry, cranberry, black currant, green tea, black tea, and many other plants. Grapeseed extract and grape skin are probably the best known sources.

Proanthocyanidins boost the antioxidant function of vitamin C. At least one study found a 1,000 percent increase in vitamin C activity. Test tube studies indicate that proanthocyanidins are 18 times more effective than vitamin C and 50 times more potent than vitamin E in neutralizing free radicals.

Proanthocyanidins are often referred to as pycnogenol. When capitalized, the term Pycnogenol refers to a patented pine bark extract. In Europe, proanthocyanidins are used in supplement form to treat weak blood capillaries (chronic venous insufficiency), post-surgical edema (swelling), cirrhosis, varicose veins, and diabetic retinopathy (damage to the eye).

Currently, pine bark extracts rich in proanthocyanidins (Pycnogenol) dominate the U.S. market. But grape skin and grapeseed extracts are equally good sources and contain another unique antioxidant (B2-3'-o-gallate) that makes them even more beneficial than the commercially available pine bark extract.

Proanthocyanidins may be particularly beneficial for people with fibromyalgia because of their effect on collagen. Collagen, the main component of connective tissue and joints, consists of twin spirals of proteins connected by cross-links. If you have joint pain it may be due to the production of too many free radicals and the release of excess amounts of an enzyme that causes the collagen in joints to become malformed. Proanthocyanidins promote healthy cartilage by normalizing collagen, and they also exert an anti-inflammatory action. This may be useful in reducing joint pain.

Physicians may prescribe proanthocyanidins therapeutically at dosages up to 300 mg per day, but most people who supplement for preventive purposes take 50 to 100 mg per day.

WATER:
THE FORGOTTEN ESSENTIAL NUTRIENT

The human body is made up of approximately 70 percent water. We can exist without food for almost five weeks, but without water, we wouldn't last more than five days. Water gives us life and keeps us alive, yet we hardly give it a thought. Water transports nutrients, regulates body temperature, and helps eliminate waste.

Being even slightly dehydrated can make you feel more fatigued. The water you drink replaces the water you lose continuously through your breath, urine, sweat, and tears. Low-level chronic dehydration, which many more people suffer than are aware, speeds the aging process and slows the body's natural abilities to detoxify and heal.

It's vitally important that you drink pure, clean water (filtered, if necessary) throughout the day, even if you don't feel thirsty. If you have poor digestion or low stomach acid, drink more water between meals and less during meals. Eight six-ounce glasses of water a day is a good average for most people. When you're sick or under extra physical or emotional stress, drink more. If you're shorter or lighter than average, you needn't force yourself to drink as much as a taller, larger person needs. A good rule of thumb is to consume 16 ounces of fluids for every 50 pounds of lean body weight. If it's hot or you are exercising and losing more fluids through perspiration, your fluid intake needs to be increased accordingly.

Plain water is best, but it's OK to substitute other beverages. Freshly juiced veggies and fruits count toward your fluids, while also helping you meet your goal of nine servings of fruits and vegetables per day.

Herbal and decaffeinated teas also count. Many teas contain folate, a B vitamin. Green tea is rich in antioxidants and may help prevent cancer. Current research suggests one or two cups of green tea per day may be beneficial. Some people say that coffee, tea, cola, and other caffeinated beverages should not count toward one's total water consumption because caffeine acts as a diuretic, causing the body to lose water. I agree that caffeine does cause you to lose a little bit of fluid, but it certainly does not eliminate a whole cup. Nevertheless, caffeine may interfere with sound sleep, so moderation is the key.

One way to make sure you drink enough fluids is to fill a pitcher or bottle with your targeted amount of water or other beverage and drink it throughout your day. Take it with you in the car and to work, or keep it nearby when you're reading or doing other activities. If the container is empty by bedtime, you've achieved your goal.

FOOD FOR THOUGHT: TWO DIETARY REGIMES TO CONSIDER

It seems you can read about a new dietary regime practically everywhere you turn. What's reliable advice, what's hearsay, and what's just another trend?

If you look to the world of complementary medicine, you'll find two time-tested dietary regimes that are based on enduring philosophies about food and lifestyle. Read more about the Ayurvedic diet and Chinese dietary therapy in Chapter 8.

Although both plans seem complex and strange to most Westerners, they have a good deal in common with the diet most American nutritionists recommend for optimal health: a plant-based diet featuring whole, unprocessed foods—whole grains, vegetables, and fruits—with some lean animal foods and some healthy fats. These dietary regimes may not only ease your fibromyalgia symptoms, they could also put you on the road to better health and help you prevent a number of diseases and chronic disorders that can hit at midlife—including high blood pressure, heart disease, and cancer.

EATING WISELY AND WELL

The foods you eat have enormous impact on your fibromyalgia symptoms and on your state of mind. Make sure you build your diet around healthy food choices by taking the following steps:

- Make food shopping trips a top priority, so you'll always have a good variety of easy-to-prepare, nutrient-rich foods on hand.
- Shop with a list.
- Emphasize vegetables and fruits, whole grains, and legumes. De-emphasize animal protein. Eat predominantly low-fat, unprocessed whole foods.
- Avoid buying high-calorie, high-fat junk foods.
- Build time into your day to prepare healthy meals for yourself.
- Freeze serving-size leftovers for days when you are too busy or too tired to cook.
- Keep healthy snacks on hand.
- Avoid, or drastically reduce, your intake of refined sugar, artificial sweeteners, hydrogenated oils, processed foods, caffeine, and alcohol.

Diet can be a critical factor in helping you manage fibromyalgia. Sticking to a nutritious diet can really pay off in terms of reduction of symptoms, more energy and vitality, and general wellness. For even more help, you'll want to boost the effects of healthy eating with supplements. You'll learn what's involved in the next chapter.

5

Taming Fibromyalgia Symptoms with Supplements and Herbs

Everything you eat, drink, and breathe impacts how good you feel and how fast you heal. As we discussed in Chapter 4, there's no single better way to boost your health than to eat and drink wholesome, nutrition-rich foods and beverages every day.

That said, we know from USDA data that about half of the U.S. population routinely eats a diet deficient in several of the basic essential nutrients (only about 60 percent of the RDA). That's the Recommended Dietary Allowances, mind you, an amount we've already identified as insufficient to promote optimal health. So diet alone is only part of the nutritional answer, particularly when it comes to the management of a complex condition like fibromyalgia.

Beyond basic good nutrition, certain nutritional supplements and herbs can supercharge your diet and help tame fibromyalgia symptoms. In this chapter we'll take a closer look at exactly which vitamins, minerals, and herbs can help ease your muscle and joint pain, promote restful sleep, lessen fatigue, reduce digestive complaints, clear "fibro-fog" (cognitive difficulties), and enhance your weakened immune system. One supplement new on the scene, S-adenosyl-methionine (SAMe), a naturally occurring amino acid found in all human tissue and organs, may offer a number of positive benefits.

As always, no advice, no matter how wise or well-intentioned, works for all of the people all of the time. Consult your physician, dietitian or nutritionist, and other practitioners in your health care team before starting any new regimen of supplements, hormones, or herbs—*especially if you are currently using any prescription medications, are receiving chemotherapy, or are under treatment for any other serious illness in addition to fibromyalgia.*

TREATING MUSCLE PAIN

Unlike the focused pain of a sprained ankle or a bump on the head, the widespread, chronic pain of fibromyalgia responds only partially to over-the-counter pain relievers. Drugs like acetaminophen and ibuprofen relieve only about 20 percent of the muscle pain associated with the disorder. That's better than nothing, but for more effective, more reliable relief, many people turn to an arsenal of pain-easing supplements and herbs.

MAGNESIUM FOR MUSCLE PAIN AND FATIGUE

The chronic muscle pain of fibromyalgia is often associated with low-level, chronic muscle tension. Therefore, anything that eases muscle tension can also relieve muscle pain. Magnesium, which is critical for transmitting nerve and muscle impulses, induces the heart muscle to relax between contractions. Found in high concentrations in the brain, blood, and bones, magnesium may help ease your muscle pain by helping chronically tensed muscles relax. It can also help increase your overall energy.

Magnesium plays a key role in the release of energy in every cell. Cells get their energy from a molecule called adenosine triphosphate (ATP), and magnesium is instrumental in creating this critical energy molecule. A recent scientific study found low levels of magnesium in the blood cells of people with fibromyalgia, helping to explain why many people with fibromyalgia feel tired much of the time.

Most people—not just those with fibromyalgia—are deficient in magnesium. Diets high in processed foods, caffeine, and sugar do not supply enough of this critical mineral for optimal health. Magnesium deficiencies are a source of many cardiovascular problems. A deficiency can also be expressed in muscle weakness and twitching, confusion, rapid heartbeat, insomnia, depression, irritability, and poor digestion. Foods high in magnesium include soy products (especially soy flour and tofu) and nuts (such as almonds, pecans, cashews, and Brazil nuts). Whole grains (particularly whole wheat, millet, and brown rice) and fruits (such as avocado and dried apricots) are other good sources. Hard water, while not ideal for your laundry, can be a valuable source.

Clinical research suggests that a combination of 300 to 600 mg of magnesium along with 1,200 to 2,400 mg of malic acid may lessen muscle pain. Taking up to 1,000 mg of magnesium per day in the form of magnesium malate will provide both nutrients in one supplement.

Magnesium can cause diarrhea in some people. Taking calcium at the same time may help. Many nutritionists suggest taking calcium and magnesium in a 2:1 ratio, such as 2,000 mg of calcium and 1,000 mg of magnesium. Dolomite and bonemeal are no longer considered good sources of magnesium and calcium because both minerals are poorly absorbed in this form and because lead has been found in these supplements.

Magnesium, like other minerals, requires some acid in the stomach for maximum absorption, so take it with meals. A bedtime dose of magnesium can help relax your muscles and ease you to sleep. If my patients are not absorbing oral magnesium adequately, I will often give them magnesium vitamin B6 shots intramuscularly, or a series of Meyer's cocktails which contain magnesium, calcium, vitamin C, and various B vitamins.

CAUTION—People with kidney disease should not take magnesium supplements without consulting a doctor.

Phenylalanine for Muscle Pain and Immunity

Phenylalanine is an essential amino acid (protein building block) found in many foods. Once absorbed by the body, it helps synthesize two key neurotransmitters: dopamine and norepinephrine. These neurotransmitters increase the level of natural pain reducers, called endorphins, in the brain. Endorphins not only relieve pain, but also may boost immunity. Recent studies have identified endorphin receptor sites on the surface of infection-fighting white blood cells. Because of the way phenylalanine acts on the central nervous system, it can decrease pain, elevate mood, enhance memory, and suppress the appetite. The recommended dosage is 1,000 mg of DL-Phenylalanine, taken twice a day on an empty stomach, 30 minutes before or two hours after a meal. This schedule aids absorption because when phenylalanine is taken between meals, it is less likely to compete with other amino acids for transport into the body's cells.

MSM (Methysulfonyl Methane) for Muscle Pain

Another supplement worth trying for pain is methysulfonyl methane (MSM). MSM is a nontoxic sulfur compound valued for its anti-inflammatory and antioxidant properties. Though more research is needed regarding its safety and actions, MSM is now available and its future appears promising. Most people take 1,000 mg per day, but therapeutic doses of up to 8,000 mg per day (in divided doses three times per day) are considered safe.

HERBS FOR PAIN:
CAPSAICIN, CURCUMIN, AND GINGER

It may surprise you to discover that several pain-relieving herbs can be found in your kitchen spice rack.

Capsaicin, the active ingredient of the herb capsicum (or cayenne red pepper), can ease muscle and joint pain. It is an ingredient in many over-the-counter external ointments developed to treat arthritis pain and muscle soreness. Zostrix is one such product available in pharmacies. Capsaicin cream causes a depletion of Substance P, a protein molecule in the nervous system that helps transmit pain impulses along nerves. Capsaicin, therefore, blocks the perception of pain. Initially, the topical application of cream can be irritating, but subsequently, as Substance P is depleted, pain gives way to relief. It may take two weeks or more to feel the full benefit of the low dose of capsicum found in over-the-counter creams. Preparations containing 0.025 to 0.075 percent capsaicin, or a cayenne tincture in the amount of 0.3 to 1 milliliter (ml) three times daily, can be used. Otherwise, follow the directions on the package.

Curcumin, the substance that gives the Indian cooking spice turmeric its yellow color, is a powerful anti-inflammatory substance that may have antioxidant properties as well. Studies show that curcumin can ease inflammation, and research indicates it may also prevent cancer in animals. Take a 500-mg capsule of curcumin powder twice a day for pain (or use it liberally in your cooking as turmeric).

Research suggests that ginger root can be an effective pain reliever because it inhibits the production of prostaglandins and leukotrienes, which are involved in pain and inflammation. For pain relief, try 1,000 mg of dried ginger twice a day, in capsules or as a tea. Use ginger with caution if you are on blood pressure or blood thinning medication or if you're scheduled for surgery or dental work; large doses of ginger can intensify the effects of such drugs and cause bleeding.

TREATING ARTHRITIS AND JOINT PAIN

People with fibromyalgia can also have symptoms from rheumatoid arthritis. Rheumatoid arthritis is a chronic disease characterized by inflammatory changes in the joints. It is thought to be an autoimmune disease, although its exact cause is not known.

Nutrition for Joint Pain

As you learned in Chapter 4, eating a nutrient-rich, plant-based diet is your best bet for health and healing. An Italian study of 46,693 people found a strong correlation between vegetable consumption and decreased incidence of rheumatoid arthritis. If you suffer from joint pain and fibromyalgia, be sure you eat five to nine servings of vegetables every day. Other studies show that following a vegan diet (plant foods only—no meat or chicken, fish, eggs, or dairy) reduces joint pain. This may be because the vegan diet eliminates those foods to which people are commonly allergic—especially eggs and dairy. It may also be because a vegan diet consists solely of whole grains, legumes, fruits, and vegetables—all high in antioxidants.

Many arthritis sufferers find that joint pain is exacerbated by certain foods. The most commonly reported triggers are dairy, corn, wheat, citrus fruits, eggs, red meat, sugar, fats, salt, and caffeine. Dairy foods are especially troublesome. You may want to try keeping a food diary and trying an elimination diet to see if any of those particular foods are problematic for you. (For advice on trying an elimination diet, see the "Food Allergies and Sensitivities" section in this chapter.) When eliminating certain foods from your diet, be sure to replace them with new types of foods to maintain variety and adequate nutrition.

METHOTREXATE FOR JOINT PAIN

The drug methotrexate is often prescribed for the treatment of rheumatoid arthritis because it suppresses an overactive immune system. Methotrexate takes the place normally held by the vitamin folic acid in an enzyme called dihydrofolate reductase, causing the B vitamin folate (or folic acid) to be lost in the urine. As mentioned previously, folate is needed for energy production and proper regulation of mood. If you have been prescribed methotrexate for joint pain, try taking extra folic acid (on the days you're not taking methotrexate) to counter the loss and help stabilize your energy and mood.

GLUCOSAMINE FOR JOINT PAIN

Glucosamine, a molecule formed from glucose (a simple sugar) and the amino acid glutamine (found naturally in muscles and joints), seems to be effective in building cartilage and thereby easing joint pain. Many people report relief from joint pain when taking 500 mg of glucosamine sulfate three times a day. Be patient; it may take from two weeks to three months to experience relief, though most people see positive effects within the first four weeks. After a few months of pain relief, try cutting back to a maintenance dose of 500 mg per day.

Cartilage extracts, although they contain glucosamine, are not recommended as a substitute for glucosamine supplements. Cartilage contains varying amounts of glucosamine and is simply a low-quality byproduct of meat production. For most people, adding chondroitin sulfate does not appear to enhance the effect of glucosamine enough to justify the added cost.

ESSENTIAL FATTY ACIDS FOR JOINT PAIN

Changing the amount and type of fat in your diet may also ease joint pain. Dietary fat affects prostaglandin metabolism, which can alter the body's immune responses, affecting autoimmune illnesses and easing joint pain. In several studies, a diet low in saturated fats, with a daily supplement of omega-3 fatty acids, decreased morning stiffness and tender joints. You can boost the amount of omega-3 in your diet by taking a fish oil supplement or adding more salmon and other cold water fish to your diet. Flaxseed is another excellent source of omega-3 fats. For tips on incorporating flaxseed into your diet, see Chapter 4.

TREATING SLEEP PROBLEMS

Most people with fibromyalgia have a rough time getting a good night's sleep. In addition to the various sleep aids and relaxation techniques available through conventional and complementary/alternative medicine, here are a few nutritional and herbal approaches worth considering.

AVOID CAFFEINE

It may seem obvious, but many people with fibromyalgia exacerbate their sleep problems by consuming caffeine during the day. Depending on how fast your body can clear the drug from your system, even one cup of coffee in the morning may keep you tossing and turning at night. Caffeine not only keeps you awake, it also works counterproductively to constrict blood vessels, contributing to headaches and muscle pain. In cases of fibromyalgia, it's generally desirable to keep blood vessels dilated (widened) to promote good circulation. When blood is circulating properly, nutrients are carried to the cells and wastes are transported away.

Caffeine also makes the adrenal glands work harder. The adrenal glands sit on top of the kidneys and produce the hormones that help the body cope with stress. Many people with fibromyalgia have "adrenal exhaustion" from chronic stress, pushing too hard and too long, and the overuse of stimulants. While the medical community recognizes Addison's disease—a condition where the adrenals are nonfunctional—marginal or sub-optimal adrenal function is a concept that is not on the radar screen of most physicians. Using coffee and other stimulants to push yourself can help you cope temporarily, but in the long run it's a strategy that does more harm than good.

If you can't or don't wish to quit consuming all caffeine, at least avoid coffee, tea, and caffeinated sodas after midday. Read food and over-the-counter medication labels for hidden caffeine. Pain relievers like Excedrin contain it, as do soft drinks like Mountain Dew, Dr. Pepper, nearly all colas, Surge, and some brands of orange soda, cream soda, and root beer. Chocolate, coffee yogurt, and coffee ice cream also contain some caffeine. Even decaffeinated coffee and tea are only 97 percent caffeine-free and can keep you awake if you're caffeine-sensitive. Add this to your growing list of good reasons to limit your intake of soda and coffee, and drink more water instead.

MELATONIN FOR SLEEP
(AND POSSIBLY DEPRESSION)

Melatonin is a naturally occurring hormone in the brain that signals the body it's time to sleep. Because melatonin is produced from serotonin, a brain chemical (neurotransmitter) that helps regulate mood, the supplement may also provide some relief from depression.

Melatonin appears to help regulate biological rhythms (sleepiness, alertness, and reaction times), keeping your "body clock" in sync. It is secreted by the pineal gland, a pea-sized gland located in the center of the brain. There is a nerve that connects the pineal gland to the eyes. When light enters the eye, it sends a signal to the pineal gland, causing it to stop producing melatonin. When evening comes, the signal stops, melatonin production resumes, and you become sleepy. In people with seasonal affective disorder (SAD), sometimes called the "winter blues," there seems to be an excess of melatonin that does not vary with the daily cycle.

If fibromyalgia is preventing you from getting a good night's rest, taking melatonin just before bed may help you get to sleep quicker and not wake as often. It is available over the counter, without prescription. You may prefer melatonin over prescription sleep aids because it is a natural product that works like the body's own sleep–wake mechanism. The recommended dosage is 1 to 3 mg, taken 60 to 90 minutes before bedtime.

You can also increase your body's own natural production of melatonin by eating bananas, barley, corn, ginger, oats, rice, and tomatoes, all of which contain small amounts of melatonin. In addition, high-carbohydrate foods can promote melatonin production when eaten in the absence of concentrated sources of protein, because in that case more of the amino acid tryptophan crosses the blood–brain barrier. Tryptophan is used to make serotonin, which is in turn made into melatonin.

Foods and beverages containing caffeine interfere with the brain's production of melatonin. Other substances—including aspirin, ibuprofen, alcohol, benzodiazepines

(Valium, Xanax), beta-blockers, calcium channel blockers, cold remedies, corticosteroids, and diuretics—also interfere with melatonin production, and so may interfere with sleep.

Melatonin is a hormone, which means that even small amounts affect several body systems as well as other hormones, such as estrogen and testosterone. Therefore, it should only be used occasionally and only after checking with your doctor.

HERBS FOR SLEEP: KAVA AND VALERIAN

If you have trouble sleeping because you need to relax, then the herb kava may be helpful. Kava (sometimes called kava kava) is used to reduce anxiety and relax muscles. Kava's active ingredients, called kava lactones, produce physical and mental relaxation and a feeling of well-being. Once you are relaxed, sleep comes more easily.

Kava is used widely in Europe for the treatment of anxiety, insomnia, and restlessness. Recent clinical studies have shown it to be as effective as prescription anxiety agents containing benzodiazepines, such as Valium. The German Commission E (akin to the U.S. Food and Drug Administration) suggests a dose of 200 to 400 mg of kava extract standardized to 30 percent kava lactones.

Because kava has few if any side effects, it is safe to use occasionally; however, it is not a supplement to be taken daily or in doses above the recommended amounts. High doses can lead to muscle weakness, visual impairment, dizziness, and skin problems. Long-term use of the herb can contribute to many problems, including liver damage. Do not combine kava with alcohol or other prescription drugs. The combination of kava and the prescription drug Xanax (alprazolam) can lead to a coma. Kava should not be used by people with Parkinson's disease, as it may interfere with dopamine.

The herb valerian can help you fall asleep more quickly and stay asleep. A mild sedative, valerian can also be used as a tranquilizer, a pain reliever, and an antispasmodic agent (relaxing the smooth muscle contractions of intestinal cramps). The herb is also helpful for relief of headaches, including migraines. In general, take one or two 150-mg capsules twice a day for anxiety, or one at bedtime to enhance sleep.

FIGHTING FATIGUE

Fatigue or low energy is one of the chief symptoms of fibromyalgia. If you feel exhausted, take it easy on yourself. Frozen foods and easy-to-prepare meals are just fine. There are many high-quality frozen foods available now, from nutritious whole wheat burritos to dinners of turkey, vegetables, and brown rice. When you do feel up to cooking, prepare more than you need and freeze the leftovers in single-serving sizes for easy reheating. Or plan meals that you assemble rather than cook. Start with previously cooked rice or grain, add frozen vegetables, some leftover cooked chicken or fish, and top with sauce from a jar for a balanced, healthy meal that won't wear you out.

If you're too tired and just don't feel like cooking, please don't reach for junk food. Your instinct may be to grab some cookies or a candy bar, but fight the urge and reach instead for some soup, half a sandwich, or even a baked potato. These choices are healthier and will give you more energy in the long run.

Several supplements can help with fatigue. We've already discussed the role of magnesium. Here are a few more to consider.

NAD (NICOTINAMIDE ADENINE DINUCLEOTIDE)

Nicotinamide adenine dinucleotide (NAD) is known to enhance energy production because, like magnesium, it helps the body create the critical energy molecule adenosine triphosphate (ATP). A recent study showed that people with chronic fatigue syndrome experienced more energy when they took NAD. The typical dose is 5 mg taken twice a day on an empty stomach.

COENZYME Q10

Coenzyme Q10 (CoQ10) is a bioenzyme also called ubiquinone, related to the word *ubiquitous*, meaning "everywhere." CoQ10 is indeed found everywhere in the body, playing a key role in the energy-producing process of every cell. If you feel low on energy, be sure you are getting enough CoQ10 so that your body has the tools it needs to make energy.

In addition to energy production, CoQ10 also functions as an antioxidant, protecting the body against chronic infections, including candida. For some fibromyalgia sufferers, it can help reduce the cognitive fuzziness known as "fibro-fog," commonly experienced during periods of flare.

Most people take 60 mg of CoQ10 twice daily for fatigue. But make sure you don't take it in the evening; you don't want to rev up right before trying to fall asleep!

DHEA

It's not uncommon for people with fibromyalgia to be physically exhausted from pushing themselves to function normally despite their illness. Eventually they run out of gas, so to speak, a condition referred to as "adrenal exhaustion." Recent research has shown that people with chronic fatigue actually have shrunken adrenal glands. Chronic stress overworks your adrenal glands, which are responsible for producing the hormone dehydroepiandrosterone (DHEA). DHEA is a precursor to many of the steroid hormones in the body, including the sex hormones. Your health care provider can test your blood or saliva for DHEA levels. Low levels have been linked to autoimmune disorders (often a side effect of the treatment), low sex drive, and exhaustion.

Use DHEA with caution. It's a powerful hormone and should only be used under the care of a physician who regularly monitors your blood levels. Too much of a good thing is as bad as not enough.

ARGININE AND ORNITHINE

Some people with fibromyalgia also show low levels of growth hormone, which like insufficient DHEA, can cause fatigue. Growth hormone shots are quite expensive. A more cost-effective alternative is to nudge the body into producing its own growth hormone by taking supplements of the amino acids arginine and ornithine.

Arginine is also important because it is a precursor to nitric oxide, which scientists have recently discovered plays a critical role in metabolism. Research involving the role of nitric oxide has led to a Nobel Prize, to important pharmaceutical products like Viagra, and to an entirely new area of research physiology. Nitric oxide dilates blood vessels, which can increase circulation in patients with fibromyalgia. The recommended dosage is 500 to 1,000 mg of a combined arginine/ornithine product taken at bedtime.

TREATING DIGESTIVE PROBLEMS

Studies have confirmed what you probably already know: Gastrointestinal disorders typically overlap with fibromyalgia. Approximately 50 to 70 percent of people with fibromyalgia have chronic stomach or digestive problems. Inadequate digestive enzymes, food allergies or sensitivities, and/or candida overgrowth may be factors to consider.

Many patients report symptoms commonly associated with a condition known as "leaky gut syndrome." In this condition, partially digested food is able to pass through the normally impermeable lining of the small intestine. The intestinal lining can be weakened by stress, toxins, chronic dietary deficiencies, and the use of nonsteroidal anti-inflammatory drugs (NSAIDs).

Proteins seem to present particular problems. The immune system, which sees the incompletely digested proteins as foreign invaders, produces antibodies which attach to the protein and can trigger a variety of undesirable immunologic reactions.

There is another negative side of leaky gut syndrome: decreased serotonin formation. Serotonin, a key neurotransmitter that figures predominantly in mood stability and sound sleep, is formed mostly in the brain and in the gastrointestinal tract.

Whatever the cause of your digestive problems, reducing or entirely eliminating animal products (red meat, chicken, eggs, etc.) from your diet and eating more vegetables can go a long way toward improving digestion. For best results, make this transition gradually but steadily. The following suggestions may also help.

TAKE A DIGESTIVE ENZYMES SUPPLEMENT

A digestive enzymes supplement can bring real relief to those with ongoing digestive problems. In order to convert food to energy, the body needs digestive enzymes. An enzyme brings molecules together in the body so a necessary chemical reaction can take place at a significantly higher rate than would occur in the absence of the enzyme. The enzyme itself is not altered in the process, so it can go on to speed up and help along additional chemical reactions.

The complete digestion of protein, fats, and carbohydrates requires digestive enzymes. Without them, the body cannot break down food so nutrients can be absorbed.

Even very small amounts of incompletely digested protein can cause profound food allergy symptoms, as we've seen in the discussion of leaky gut syndrome. Partially digested fat is not believed to cause allergic reactions, but it does contribute to impaired fat absorption, meaning the body has trouble absorbing the fat-soluble vitamins A, D, E, and K and the essential fatty acids. Partially digested carbohydrates may be fully digested later by the "friendly bacteria" living in the intestinal tract, but the result is gas, bloating, and cramping.

To assure proper digestion, take one or two capsules of mixed digestive enzymes (including papain, bromelain, and betaine) with each meal.

UNDERSTAND ALLERGIES AND SENSITIVITIES

Whether attributable to a lack of digestive enzymes or to some other cause, food allergies and/or sensitivities can cause serious problems for people with fibromyalgia. Food allergies occur when the body's immune system misreads a particular food or ingredient as a threat to the body and, as a result, produces antibodies to that food. The next time that food is eaten, the immune system reacts as if a virus or other disease-causing agent has invaded the body and it launches an attack.

Food allergies are different from respiratory allergies, and those who have them express a wider range of symptoms. People with food allergies or sensitivities may experience nausea, diarrhea, scratchy skin, rashes, hives, headaches, congestion, joint and muscle aches, watery eyes, and/or sore throat. Emotional symptoms are common and include fatigue, cognitive fog, mood swings, and insomnia. The role of food allergies and sensitivities is a controversial topic within medical circles. Many physicians are totally closed to this possibility.

Altogether, more than 160 different foods are recognized allergens. Ninety percent of all food allergies and sensitivities are caused by just a handful of foods. Some of the more common culprits include: chocolate, citrus, coconut, coffee, corn, cow's milk, eggs, fish, mustard, peanuts, peas, pork, shellfish, soybeans, tomatoes, tree nuts, wheat, and yeast. Some people outgrow food allergies acquired in childhood, only to acquire new sensitivities as adults.

Dear Diary

If you suspect you are allergic to any food or have problems with your digestive system, the best way to track down the culprits is to keep a food diary. Writing down everything you eat and any symptoms you experience can help you and your doctor sort out possible food sensitivities.

The operative word here is *everything*. Write down everything you eat and drink every day for a week. Break out mixed food into its components. If you feel poorly after eating stew you need to know all of the ingredients to determine if it was the meat, carrots, or wheat flour that was the problem. A few visits to a registered dietitian who specializes in allergies can help you with this detective work.

Many food sensitivities found in people with fibromyalgia are not the type to cause emergency symptoms, as is the case with people who eat, for example, a peanut and must seek immediate medical attention. With fibromyalgia, most food allergies are the delayed hypersensitivity type; the negative reaction to an offending food may not occur for hours. That makes your detective work harder, but well worth the effort.

If you suspect multiple allergies or are just not sure what might be causing the problem, your health care professional may suggest a strict elimination diet to help with diagnosis. Start on a bland diet of mostly rice, apple juice, and turkey for a couple of days. Then slowly add back foods to which you think you are not allergic, one at a time, recording any adverse reactions. Next, try a food that you suspect you may be allergic to, again recording any reactive symptoms. The key to surviving the elimination diet is to eat enough food. The first few days you'll be eating a lot of turkey and rice. Hang in there; it won't last forever.

Once you discover which food or foods aggravate your condition, you must eliminate them from your diet. Read labels carefully to avoid ingesting any allergen that is an ingredient in a prepared or processed food.

The next step is to focus on foods to add back to your diet. If you need to avoid dairy, be sure to add nondairy sources of calcium like green leafy vegetables and calcium-fortified orange juice. If you need to eliminate wheat, make up the deficit with other grains like quinoa, amaranth, and brown rice. For more information on this topic, contact the Food Allergy Network at *www.foodallergy.org* or call 800-929-4040.

DEALING WITH DYSBIOSIS

Dysbiosis is the term used to describe an imbalance in the type and amount of bacteria normally present in the intestines. This imbalance can make you feel ill and cause a variety of chemical and immune problems. To correct dysbiosis, take a probiotic supplement of "good bacteria," such as *Lactobacillus acidophilus,* or eat food with active bacteria cultures, like yogurt. Good bacteria help crowd out and generally make conditions unfavorable for disease-causing "bad bacteria."

Taking a prebiotic supplement (one that feeds the good bacteria already living in your intestines) along with the probiotic will increase its effectiveness. It's like fertilizing your garden to promote plant growth. The most common prebiotic is fructooligosaccharide (FOS). FOS is a naturally occurring substance consisting of short chains of fructose (fruit sugar). Take 1 to 4 grams a day, with your supplemental probiotic.

Both prebiotic and probiotic supplements have a number of positive health benefits. They reduce the production of toxic and cancer-causing compounds in the intestinal tract. Good bacteria make short-chain fatty acids (SCFA). These make the colon slightly acidic, which helps destroy bad bacteria. This acidity aids the absorption of minerals like magnesium. Short-chain fatty acids also directly feed the cells of the intestine and help keep them healthy. This is especially important for people experiencing ongoing digestive problems.

When taking *Lactobacillus acidophilus,* start with one capsule per day for two weeks, then increase to two capsules per day for two weeks, and then cut back to one capsule per day. Use only fresh, living, refrigerated acidophilus preparations.

There is controversy as to whether acidophilus should be taken with meals. While there may be some advantages to taking acidophilus or other probiotics between meals, I think it makes life more complicated than it needs to be. For this reason, I generally suggest taking it with a meal, along with any other supplements you take. If you have to hire a secretary to remind you when to take your supplements, your routine is too complicated!

CANDIDA OVERGROWTH SYNDROME

Another type of dysbiosis is caused by the overgrowth of a naturally occurring yeast called candida. Candida is present in all of us, and it is generally kept under control by friendly bacteria in the intestine. We're usually never even aware of it. However, sometimes the candida organisms reach a level where they migrate outside the intestine. This sometimes follows a course of treatment with antibiotics which kill off some of the friendly bacteria, along with the germs they are supposed to attack. This gives the candida an opportunity to proliferate.

Many people with fibromyalgia have excessive levels of candida (as determined by either blood testing or stool cultures). This can lead to nausea, headaches, depression, abnormal fatigue, and other problems common to fibromyalgia patients. Candida overgrowth syndrome is a controversial diagnosis that most doctors don't believe in. I didn't believe in it myself until I started ordering the tests. Repeatedly seeing patients with abnormally elevated candida tests respond to antifungal treatments (with corresponding improvements in their test results) has convinced me that for some patients candida overgrowth is a legitimate diagnosis. Unfortunately, the research needed to adequately prove or disprove this syndrome has not been done yet. Does a tree falling in the forest make any noise if there is nobody there to hear it? Does candida overgrowth actually exist if the medical community doesn't do the tests and research to prove it? In the meantime, until the diagnosis of candida overgrowth is given the official blessing of the medical establishment, there are several things you can do.

Probiotics and prebiotics can be useful in such cases. Some physicians may prescribe antifungal medications, like Nystatin, or suggest an "anti-candida diet." This is a very restrictive diet that requires avoiding all sugars, many carbohydrates (including bread and fruit), all yeast-containing foods, all fermented products, mushrooms, and vinegar. The principle here is "don't feed the yeast." The problem is, most people following such a drastic diet focus on what *not* to eat and end up not eating enough to maintain proper nutrition.

I take a more moderate approach. The human body runs on a sugar called glucose, so you cannot starve candida out of your body. But you can avoid providing a "feast for the yeast" by cutting way back on the refined sugar in your diet. Do this by eliminating between-meal sodas, juices, candies, sweets, and any snacks made with sugar, sucrose, fructose, glucose, dextrose, maltose, or any of the "oses" listed on the product label. Have an occasional sweet *with a meal* if you must; the negative effects of the sugar are diluted by the other foods you're digesting at the same time.

Candida cannot be totally eliminated, nor should it be. The purpose of candida treatment is to achieve an acceptable balance of all the organisms living in the body, and to make your digestive tract an inhospitable host, discouraging candida overgrowth.

BOOSTING IMMUNITY

While no one can pinpoint exactly what causes fibromyalgia, immune system problems likely play a key role. Recurrent colds, chronic sinus or skin infections, and hidden dental infections can linger for years, eroding your overall health.

In addition to improving immune function with antioxidants, it can be helpful to supplement with colostrum and ginseng, especially if you are experiencing repeated or lingering infections. Be sure to talk to your doctor about any acute infections, as well as any low-grade infection that keeps coming back.

GINSENG

There are three types of ginseng available today: Asian, Siberian, and American. All have somewhat similar effects on the body. Ginseng can be helpful in reducing the effects of stress, and it can boost energy levels, enhance memory, and stimulate the immune system. Ginseng's main active ingredients are compounds called ginsenosides, which neutralize the effects of stress on the body. Animal studies have shown consistently that ginseng is an effective immune booster.

For added energy and to enhance immunity, try a cup or two of ginseng tea daily. Alternately, take 10 to 40 drops of ginseng tincture mixed in warm water, or 500 mg of a ginseng supplement twice a day. Don't take ginseng at night, as it may interfere with sound sleep. Also be cautious with ginseng supplements if you have high blood pressure.

COLOSTRUM

Colostrum is the clear, thin "premilk" that mammals produce for their infants before the regular milk begins to flow. Colostrum contains antibodies that kill off viruses and bacteria and transfer passive immune factors to the animal or person consuming it. People with fibromyalgia who suffer from recurrent infections may benefit from these passive immune factors, and even patients who are allergic to dairy products are often able to tolerate colostrum. Try 2,000 mg twice daily if you experience recurrent infections. Unlike echinacea or astralagus (which are immune stimulants), colostrum seems to provide more passive immunity. In patients with autoimmune disease, immune stimulants can worsen their illness. Colostrum, because it works through more passive mechanisms, appears to be well tolerated even by patients with autoimmune disease.

A NEW ADDITION TO THE
FIBROMYALGIA ARSENAL:
S-ADENOSYL-METHIONINE (SAMe)

The supplement S-adenosyl methionine (SAMe, pronounced "Sammy") has been available by prescription for many years in Europe, where doctors prescribe it for depression, fibromyalgia, osteoarthritis, and chronic fatigue syndrome. Most people who take it report an increase in concentration, energy, alertness, and well-being.

The compound is made from the amino acid methionine. SAMe works by influencing the formation of brain chemicals and by helping preserve glutathione, an important antioxidant. It is involved in more than 35 different bodily processes—including helping the body maintain cell membranes and removing toxic substances.

Most important for people with depression—and that includes many fibromyalgia sufferers—SAMe makes brain cells more responsive to the neurotransmitters that regulate mood, such as serotonin. Neurotransmitters need a place to attach to brain cells before they can pass along the message to feel better. These attachment points, called receptors, float on the membranes of brain cells like water lilies on a pond. If the cell coating becomes thick and gluey due to age, a diet high in saturated fats, or other problems, the receptors lose their ability to help pass along chemical signals. SAMe prevents the membranes from becoming sticky and helps keep the receptors ready for action.

For this reason, SAMe appears to be a very effective antidepressant. In 14 countries it is considered a prescription drug, and doctors around the world have used it to treat depression for over 20 years. Since the 1970s, the results of 40 clinical studies involving roughly fourteen hundred patients have been published in the scientific literature. In one study, researchers at the University of California at Irvine gave 17 severely depressed patients a four-week course of SAMe or desipramine, a prescription antidepressant. The SAMe recipients had a slightly higher response rate (62 percent) than the people on desipramine (50 percent). The findings of all of the 40 trials consistently showed that SAMe works about as well as prescription antidepressants, and it's clearly less toxic, meaning fewer side effects. Other than nausea, SAMe doesn't seem to cause major adverse effects, even at high doses. Studies do suggest, however, that just like other antidepressants, SAMe may trigger manic episodes in people with bipolar disorder, so this is not the treatment of choice for that condition.

There is a secondary benefit with SAMe, one of particular interest to people with fibromyalgia: relief from the symptoms of arthritis. Some of the first people who were given SAMe for depression also suffered joint pain from osteoarthritis. SAMe provided relief for both conditions. It seems that when the body is done using a molecule of SAMe in the brain, it breaks it down into sulfur-containing compounds that move through the blood to the joints where they help maintain joint cartilage. SAMe also plays a role in the formation of myelin, the protective white sheath that surrounds nerve cells like the insulation on a wire.

The body manufactures SAMe from the amino acid methionine, found in soybeans, eggs, seeds, lentils, and meat. However, a deficiency of vitamin B_{12} or folic acid can disrupt production. Supplementing directly with methionine is not the way to increase SAMe, since high doses can be toxic and do not seem to increase body levels of SAMe.

The recommended dose is 400 mg three to four times daily. SAMe can cause nausea and gastrointestinal disturbances in some people, so it's a good idea to start at a dose of 200 mg twice daily, then increase gradually. At the recommended doses, SAMe can be very expensive. As the use of this supplement becomes more widespread, the economic law of supply and demand should bring its price down to a more reasonable and affordable range.

6

You Are How You Live: Lifestyle Strategies for Feeling Better

No matter *what* life throws your way, the most important factor in determining your well-being is not your illness, your doctor, your treatments, or your support team. It's you. Every day, the things you do and don't do, eat and don't eat, think and don't think significantly affect your health. While there are certainly factors outside your control, how you choose to live ultimately shapes the quality of your life. The downside is there's no one else to blame if your symptoms flare. The upside is that *you*— not the latest drug or the newest technology—have the power to change how you feel.

If you suffer from fibromyalgia and you want to feel better, there are dozens of ways to take control of your life. I have discussed ways you can better understand fibromyalgia, find the right doctor, get an accurate diagnosis, and triage your conventional treatment options. Now, before we discuss the bounty of complementary and alternative medical approaches, let's focus on the many things you can do, on your own, to make your life better. These include:

- Continuing to learn about fibromyalgia
- Committing yourself to moderate exercise, good posture, and great nutrition
- Avoiding environmental toxins
- Quitting smoking, limiting alcohol, and dealing with addictions
- Coping with stress and depression
- Dealing with family, children, marriage, and intimacy
- Understanding your rights at work and school

STAY IN THE PILOT'S SEAT

Despite its great accomplishments, a profound shortcoming of conventional Western medicine is its tacit assumption that the patient will take a passive role in the process. While this expectation works quite well if you are wheeled into a hospital emergency room on a stretcher, it's not particularly useful in the ongoing management of chronic illnesses. Coping successfully with disorders like fibromyalgia requires that you get involved and stay involved. I cannot overstate how crucial this is for your maximum comfort and good health.

To stay in the pilot's seat, learn all you can about the collection of symptoms we call fibromyalgia. Take notes or make tape recordings of all health care consultations and keep copies of all your lab test results. Ask a lot of questions and be completely candid when questions are asked of you. Choose less aggressive treatments first unless the situation is dangerous, and aggressive (more risky) interventions absolutely necessary. Inform your physician of all medications, herbal remedies, and nutritional supplements you take or are considering taking. Keep a journal of your symptoms and triggers, and give treatments time to work before seeking relief elsewhere.

Stay in charge, informed, and positive. Expect success. While there's no cure for fibromyalgia, there's every reason to expect to feel better.

EXERCISE: MOVING TOWARD RELIEF

Moving your body may seem like the *last* thing you want or should do, but the muscle pain of fibromyalgia often greatly diminishes with moderate exercise.

When muscles hurt, other muscles compensate. This works for a while, but then the compensating muscles start hurting, too. The more pain you feel, the less you move. In time, lack of exercise causes muscles to decondition, becoming smaller and weaker. Weak muscles easily become painful muscles, which leads to more compensation, followed by even more inactivity, and . . . well, you get the picture. Exercise is vital to the successful management of fibromyalgia because it breaks this debilitating cycle.

In addition to easing pain by building and toning your muscles, exercise strengthens the heart, improves circulation, and helps keep bones strong. Regular exercise lowers excessive cholesterol. And studies show that regular physical exercise can boost energy during the day and help you to sleep better at night. Exercise can even help relieve depression and anxiety by releasing endorphins, your body's natural painkillers that also promote a sense of well-being.

Before beginning any exercise program, consult your doctor. People with fibromyalgia often require special precautions when exercising. For instance, athletic shoes need to fit properly, with flexible soles and good, even support through the whole foot (check for signs of uneven wear along the soles). If you enjoy the water, exercising in a pool is great because the pressure of the water helps cushion sore muscles and supports you from all sides. But make sure the pool is heated to a fairly warm 88 to 94 degrees Fahrenheit. Exposure to colder water temperatures may worsen your fibromyalgia symptoms.

Pick exercises you actually enjoy. Countless people embark on programs of exercise, only to abandon them shortly afterward. Studies show that many exercise "dropouts" chose exercises they didn't like. If you don't like running, don't run. If you hate getting wet, don't swim. Forget aerobics if you think you'll look undignified or silly. Give some serious thought to choosing a fun exercise you will enjoy.

Don't buy expensive equipment until you are sure you like the exercise. How can you be sure you'll like a stair-climber or a stationary bike before you buy it? Most reputable stores will allow you to test equipment. Visit the store in exercise clothes, prepared for a workout. If the thought of exercising in a store embarrasses you, visit a gym or ask a friend if you can try her equipment. Don't fall into the trap of furnishing your basement and garage with unused exercise machines. We could probably eliminate the national budget deficit if everyone would sell their unused exercise equipment and donate the money to the government. The only problem with this is that the same exercise equipment would now gather dust in a different set of basements and garages.

Consider asking a family member or friend to start an exercise program with you. When you exercise with a partner, you are more likely to continue. A partner can help to motivate you. It's a lot tougher to break a commitment to someone you care about than to skip a solo workout.

Start your exercise program *slowly and gently*. Give your body time to adapt to the new demands you're placing on it. Set realistic goals and don't do too much too soon. It's common for people with fibromyalgia to overexert themselves when they have a good day, injure themselves, and then feel like they've been run over by a truck a few hours or a few days later. People who exceed their limitations sooner or later become frustrated and give up. If you've lived with fibromyalgia for a long time without exercising, your muscles are most likely weak and uncoordinated. Certain muscles may have modified their actions to compensate for other muscles that are less functional. It will take some time to bring your body back to improved functioning, but it will be worth the wait. When exercising, remember the patient, persistent tortoise who won the race.

Here are some tips for a successful exercise program:

- Warm up and stretch first. Never exercise when your muscles are cold or tired. Fifteen minutes of warm up prepares your muscles for exertion. Follow with 10 minutes of gentle stretching to improve flexibility and range of motion.
- Schedule your workouts for when you feel your best during the day. For many people with fibromyalgia, this is between 10:00 A.M. and 2:00 P.M.
- Avoid exercising in hot or cold temperatures.
- Replenish body fluids frequently during your workout, consuming at least eight ounces of water for every 15 minutes of exercise, regardless of your thirst.
- Consider an exercise plan that incorporates more than one type of workout. For example, walk on Monday, practice yoga on Tuesday, and lift light weights on Wednesday. That way you'll avoid overworking particular muscles, minimize boredom, and you will work different parts of your body in different ways. This will also give you alternatives to being sidelined because of bad weather or a closed gym.
- When you're done, stretch gently again, while muscles are warm and loose.

It's particularly important for people with consistent pain in certain tender or trigger points to take special precautions with repetitive exercises that constantly stress the same muscle groups. This would include such mundane tasks as vacuuming, sweeping, raking, shoveling snow, or even unloading the dishwasher. If you perform these tasks, try to vary your movements, switching sides every six or seven repetitions so you're alternating muscle groups with pauses in between to allow muscles to rest.

Your health care providers can suggest some exercise activities that take your symptoms into account. Try to include *aerobic, flexibility, and strengthening exercises* in any workout program.

AEROBIC EXERCISES

The mere mention of aerobic exercise leaves many of us imagining an energetic, fit woman in colorful spandex, cheerfully leading a group of people through a series of bouncy exercises to rhythmic music. But that's just one type of aerobic exercise.

Aerobic, or endurance, exercise refers to any exercise where both your respiration and heart rate become elevated. During an aerobic workout, your body uses oxygen from the air you breathe to help your cells and tissues manage the stress of exercising. Aerobic exercise conditions your heart and lungs to make them more efficient. It can also be helpful for weight loss, weight control, creating a feeling of well-being, and improving sleep.

Dancing, swimming, bicycling, or walking at a rapid pace are all recommended. Avoid any exercise, like step aerobics, that requires bouncing, as this could force muscles to stretch beyond their limit.

FLEXIBILITY EXERCISES

Flexibility or range-of-motion exercises are designed to improve the mobility of joints and loosen tight muscles, tendons, and ligaments. People with fibromyalgia and other chronic conditions often attempt to deal with painful muscles by not using them. This eventually results in even tighter muscles and stiffer joints. Flexibility exercises are designed to reverse this decline with the ultimate goal of relieving pain. Try to exercise both sides of your body equally to maintain good balance.

Ask a physical therapist or other exercise professional to show you some flexibility exercises. For best results, do your routine daily. Everyday tasks, such as vacuuming or stair climbing, are no substitutes for workouts that focus on improving your range of motion.

STRENGTHENING EXERCISES

Strengthening exercises help to maintain or increase muscle strength. Stronger muscles are much more effective at supporting the body and helping you cope with the painful effects of fibromyalgia. Strengthening exercises can be either *isometric* or *isotonic*.

Isometric exercises allow you to tighten your muscles without moving your joints. Think of a cartoon muscle man flexing his biceps to impress someone, and you've got the idea. Isometric exercise is useful if you must avoid using painful joints. Isotonic exercises require the movement of joints to strengthen muscles. For example, if you were seated in a chair and lifted your lower leg, you would be working the large muscle group on the front of your upper leg. Both isometric and isotonic exercises are useful for people with fibromyalgia because they can be performed while sitting, reclining, or standing. This reduces strain on painful joints and muscles.

If you're incorporating some weight-bearing, bone-strengthening exercises into your routine (important for the prevention of osteoporosis), start out gradually. Begin with a weight you can lift 10 times without strain, with the last two repetitions becoming more difficult. For some people, this may be one or two pounds; others may start out with 15- to 20-pound weights. As your muscles become stronger, and as long as you're not experiencing pain, increase the weights in one- and two-pound increments.

Don't Forget to Breathe!

Proper breathing is beneficial during all types of exercise. Because breathing is automatic, few of us ever think about how to breathe properly. Unfortunately, many of us develop bad habits; but with practice, they can be overcome. Proper inhaling first fills the abdomen, then the middle chest, and finally, the upper chest. This is in sharp contrast to our image of correct posture: stomach in, chest out. Instead, we should relax our abdominal muscles and lift our chests to fill our lungs completely, allowing our diaphragm to do most of our breathing, and resulting in a deeper, more healthful exchange of air.

During exercise, you want to increase your air intake. Pay attention to your breathing while you exercise; try to prevent it from becoming quick and shallow. Practice proper breathing at rest, later incorporating it into your exercise routine. In general, you should breathe in through your nose and out through your mouth when exercising.

POSTURE

Another body process most of us don't think about at all is our maintenance of body position, or posture. As with breathing, poor posture habits develop over time and require conscious, sustained effort to change.

Check your posture frequently. Fibromyalgia patients often stand with their heads forward, their shoulders rounded and elevated, and their knees hyper-extended. They also bear more weight on one leg than the other. When standing, keep your weight balanced evenly between both feet, which should be spread about a shoulder-width apart. Relax your shoulders and lift your chest. Try to avoid habits like hunching forward while sitting.

Physical therapist Janet Hulme recommends practicing the following steps until proper posture becomes second nature:

While standing:
- Distribute your weight equally between both feet.
- Unlock your knees.
- Center your pelvis over your knees and feet.

- Lift your chest up and out.
- Release your shoulders.
- Release your jaw, and keep your teeth apart and your tongue released from the roof of your mouth.
- Hold your head back with your chin dropped slightly.
- Lengthen your spine by imagining a string attached to the top of your head, pulling you upward.

While sitting:
- Distribute your weight equally between both hips.
- Center your pelvis over your hips.
- Lift your chest up and out.
- Release your shoulders.
- Release your jaw, and keep your teeth apart and your tongue released from the roof of your mouth.
- Hold your head back with your chin dropped slightly.
- Lengthen your spine by imagining a string attached to the top of your head, pulling you upward.
- Slowly breathe from your lower abdomen.

While bending:
- Never lift, bend, or twist at the same time.
- Turn your feet in the direction you want to bend.
- Look up before you bend. This will help your spine align properly.

Ask your physical therapist for recommendations about good body posture and devote time to practicing these techniques. You may want to look for a practitioner who can train you in the Alexander technique or the Feldenkrais method, two therapies that emphasize proper body mechanics. Learn more about them in Chapter 11.

EATING FOR HEALTH AND HAPPINESS

A full serving of vital nutrition information was offered in Chapters 4 and 5. Here are a few healthy nibbles to remember as you take charge of your health:

- Eat whole, high-quality, nutrition-dense foods—especially fresh vegetables, fruits, whole grains, and legumes.
- Limit or avoid animal foods, such as red meat, chicken, and eggs.
- Avoid foods that have been extensively processed.
- Avoid artificial sweeteners and limit refined sugars.
- Strive for balance, variety, and pleasure. Try new tastes, but don't eat what you don't like.
- Eat under relaxed circumstances. Savor each bite.
- Listen to your body. Stop eating when you feel full.

AVOIDING ENVIRONMENTAL TOXINS

In today's polluted and chemical-filled world, it's impossible to avoid coming into daily contact with environmental toxins, including car exhaust, secondhand smoke, lead paint, and pesticides. Even medications, noise, light, and scents can irritate you and trigger (or aggravate) your symptoms.

People with fibromyalgia are sometimes highly sensitive to common substances that don't seem to affect other people. Reactions to such irritants can run the gamut from fatigue, aches, irritability, hives, and drowsiness to the rarer experience of systemwide shock. Because many symptoms of chemical sensitivity can be similar to those of fibromyalgia, you may need a physician's help to identify possible culprits. Your doctor may recommend an elimination protocol, in which you remove certain substances from your diet or environment for two to six weeks, and then reintroduce them, one at a time.

If sensitivities to common substances are bothering you but are not incapacitating, try the following measures before starting a full-blown elimination protocol:

- Avoid toxic or harsh cleaners and other chemicals at home, work, and school. Many nontoxic alternatives work equally well. Check your local health food store or a good supermarket for a selection of natural or "green" products, including window spray, toilet cleaner, laundry detergent, bath soap, deodorant, shampoo, and toothpaste.
- Whenever possible, eat organic fruits and vegetables that are pesticide-free or pesticide-reduced. Avoid food grown or prepared in other countries, like Mexico, where fewer laws protect the food supply. Wash commercially grown produce with a

citrus-based fruit and vegetable wash to reduce surface pesticides. If symptoms persist, try eliminating common allergy-causing foods, such as milk, wheat, eggs, citrus, and chocolate, or see your physician or allergist for specific testing.

- Eliminate or reduce your consumption of artificial sweeteners (Nutrasweet and Equal), hydrogenated oils (found in many processed foods), and refined sugar.

- Eliminate or reduce your exposure to electromagnetic fields (EMFs). Sensitivity to EMFs is common among people with fibromyalgia, possibly because EMFs adversely affect activity in the autonomic nervous system. Flares seem to increase sensitivity. A Russian study found 25 percent of those studied were electromagnetically sensitive.

The role of electromagnetic fields in health is hotly debated, but it appears that EMFs can have both good and bad effects. In general, an alternating current (AC) electromagnetic field (the kind produced by power lines, fluorescent lighting, electric blankets, and most electrical appliances) tends to have a negative effect because it interferes with the body's electrical activity, which is, for the most part, direct current (DC). Have you ever held up a radio to your computer screen or TV screen? The static or distortion is caused by EMF interference (two incompatible electromagnetic fields). It's similar to the physiologic "static" or "distortion" experienced by EMF-sensitive individuals upon exposure to alternating current

EMFs. On the other hand, some EMFs (those that *are* compatible with electrical activity in the body) may have favorable effects.

A 1995 study revealed that some groups of people are particularly reactive to certain winds high in EMF activity. Such positively-charged winds (including the Sirocco in Italy, the Chinook in the Rocky Mountains, and the Santa Ana in California) were shown to increase serotonin levels. Many people with fibromyalgia have low levels of serotonin, and atmospheric conditions might help them feel better by boosting this neurotransmitter.

If you have an EMF sensitivity, alert your health care team. This is an important symptom, and something to keep in mind when developing your treatment strategy. In the meantime, limit your exposure to electromagnetic fields and avoid fluorescent lighting if possible. Some people with fibromyalgia try to avoid electric blankets, waterbed heaters, hair dryers, and other electric items. Keep computer use to a minimum, especially during a flare.

There's no point in worrying about every possible environmental hazard everywhere you go. But at least in your own home (and perhaps even at work, if you can arrange it), try to limit your exposure to toxins. Of special importance is the bedroom. This is the room where we spend most of our time, and it should be the most environmentally safe. Here are a few ideas to consider:

- Never leave cleaning fluids or containers in your bedroom.
- Check for moldy books and dusty book shelves.

- Vacuum the carpet regularly—or better yet, get rid of it! It's full of dead skin cells, along with dust mites and their excrement. All of these substances can aggravate allergies.
- New carpeting and new mattresses can release chemicals into your bedroom air for several weeks. Leave new beds in another room or in the garage until they air out. If your new carpet has a chemical odor, leave your windows open or sleep elsewhere for a while.

If your doctor or other health care providers suspect you may be chemically sensitive, learn more about your particular condition and needs. You may find it helpful, for example, to ask someone else to pump gas into your car for you so you don't have to breathe the hydrocarbons. Or you may wish to avoid salad bars in restaurants if the lettuce is sprayed with a chemical to keep it looking fresh. There are many excellent books with advice on how to make your home or workplace less irritating.

QUIT SMOKING, LIMIT ALCOHOL, AND DEAL WITH ADDICTIONS

I won't mince words. If you smoke, quit. If you drink too much, cut back. And if drug addiction has taken hold of your life, get help.

Nicotine is not just habit-forming, it's a deadly poison. Nicotine in cigarettes causes blood vessels to constrict, decreasing the flow of blood, oxygen, and nutrients to your muscles, and increasing pain and muscle tension. In addition, smoking may actually increase your already high levels of Substance P, that bothersome natural compound that heightens our perception of pain. Nicotine also causes the autonomic nervous system to function abnormally, which increases the likelihood that you'll experience sensations of burning, numbness, and tingling. Smoking is just bad news for people with fibromyalgia.

Kicking the habit is a whole lot easier said than done. If you just can't seem to quit smoking, ask your physician for help. Acupuncture and/or herbal preparations have helped some people give up cigarettes. Nicotine gum or patches can help you get past the rough spots. Support groups help some people; others prefer to go it alone. Once you're smoke-free, you'll reap immediate health benefits, including less pain and a lower risk of heart disease, cancer, and other illnesses.

If you consume alcohol, do so in very limited amounts, and refrain from drinking on a daily basis. Alcohol is a depressant and can intensify many fibromyalgia symptoms. Develop other, more effective ways to relax. (See the section "Soothing Stress," which follows.)

If you use illicit drugs or are addicted to any substance or medication, please tell your physician. Even if you're not ready to change your habits, your doctor needs to know what's going into your body so he or she can best guide your treatment. Contrary to stereotypic images, the average drug addict looks just like you or me and is a fully employed, normal-looking, contributing member of society who desperately needs help—but isn't ready for it or doesn't know how to get it. You needn't go to a drug treatment clinic if that intimidates you. You can get private help from many physicians, and there are countless Twelve-Step programs and other similar programs to support you. Pain of all kinds drives people into addictions. If you are one of those individuals, get the help you deserve.

SOOTHING STRESS

We hear the word stress everywhere we turn, and we've built a whole vocabulary around the concept. We say we're "stressed" when we feel agitated or overwhelmed. We may attribute overreactions to being "stressed out," and we talk about hobbies and exercise in terms of "stress reduction." But few of us understand what stress really means.

Stress is anything that tends to push our minds and/or our bodies out of the homeostatic comfort zone. When we find ourselves in situations we *perceive* as dangerous, a set of chemical and physiologic reactions are triggered. Our bodies are hard-wired for survival. When we perceive we are threatened, our bodies automatically prepare us to take some kind of action. Our heart rate and rate of respiration increase and our blood pressure rises. These and other physiological changes prepare us for "fight or flight." We are ready—in an instant—to fight off our attacker or run from danger as quickly as possible.

The trouble is that we are fully capable of jumping into survival mode without a true threat. Getting cut off by another car on the highway, for example, can trigger the same stress response as coming face to face with a tiger: heart rate increases, breathing quickens, and blood pressure rises. In addition, stress responses are supposed to last only long enough for the immediate danger to pass, enabling us, for example, to climb a tree and avoid being eaten by that tiger. But too often in today's world, our stress responses become chronic. It's like we're pushing our own internal panic button over and over, rather than once in a blue moon to save ourselves from a truly life-threatening danger.

In a very real sense, you control your own stress level. Even though many situations are external to us and are not within our control, we *can* control the way we perceive and respond to those external situations. If you allow yourself to get angry every time you're cut off by another driver, you—not the other guy—are creating the stress. Even if you constantly see red when driving in traffic, you can make a conscious effort to calm down and prevent a stress response.

Chronic stress responses can have serious health effects, including headache, stomach problems, high blood pressure, muscle tension (including backache), fatigue, irritability, eating disorders, mood disorders, and compromised immune system function. Many of the characteristics of fibromyalgia—impaired physical function, chronic pain, and an uncertain future—are themselves significant stressors. It is therefore especially important for those with fibromyalgia to learn how to reduce stress and control their chronic stress response.

A recent survey revealed that 63 percent of fibromyalgia sufferers feel that stress plays a major role in influencing their symptoms and the course of their disease. Your body has a specific set of responses to stress. The key to keeping your stress at a manageable level is to make these responses work *for* you, not against you. The following techniques may help:

- Each individual's chronic stress response can produce a unique set of problems. Learn to recognize your body's particular stress signals.
- Identify those situations and people that trigger your stress reaction. Until you can "reprogram" yourself, consider avoiding these triggers whenever possible. You can't avoid every stressor, but you don't have to invite them into your life.
- Find ways to accept and manage the stressful situations you cannot eliminate. Don't waste energy trying to change people or situations over which you have no control. Accept what you can't change and move on. Forgive anyone whom you feel has wronged you. Holding on to resentments and grudges only hurts you—not the other person. Sometimes taking charge means *letting go*.
- Be flexible. Your condition demands it!
- Lower your standards and expectations. Let the dishes sit for a while longer, clean your house less frequently, wear clothes that are truly comfortable, use gift bags instead of wrapping paper, don't drive at rush hour, and delegate tasks to others.

- Set aside time to relax every day, no matter what.
- Communicate your needs directly. You have that right.
- Develop a hobby. Engaging in something you enjoy relieves stress and gives you a creative outlet.
- Pace yourself. Don't try to do too much in an unrealistic time frame. Prioritize. Break down big tasks into manageable pieces. Start early and don't rush. For example, start your Christmas shopping during the midsummer sales.
- Simplify. Get rid of things you don't use regularly. Find ways to do tasks more efficiently. Set realistic goals. Use the time you save to pamper yourself.
- Experiment with mind–body therapies. Try to reduce stress using guided imagery, prayer, soft music, being with friends, or deep breathing. You'll find lots of useful information in Chapter 12.

DEALING WITH DEPRESSION

There are times when each of us feels blue, inadequate, or overwhelmed. But when feelings of profound sadness or hopelessness become aspects of daily living, you are depressed and need help.

Unfortunately, depression and fibromyalgia often go hand in hand. More than two dozen studies have focused on depression in people with fibromyalgia. According to these studies, approximately one out of five fibromyalgia patients could be identified as severely depressed at the time of their office visit. And more than half have a history of major depression at some time in their lives.

Depression, major or not, can be a big roadblock on your route to feeling better. Regardless of severity or frequency, depression calls for *action*. The first step is to recognize the disorder. Signs of depression may include some or all of the following, when present for at least two weeks:

- Sleeping too much or too little.
- Diminished interest in daily activities.
- Loss of concentration or an inability to process information.
- Loss of interest in life and in the activities and people you usually enjoy.
- Overwhelming feelings of sadness, guilt, or worthlessness nearly every day.
- Lack of interest in sex.
- Major changes in eating habits, either eating too much or too little.
- Thoughts of suicide or attempts to commit suicide.

There are several kinds of depression, each with a range of possible causes and potential treatments. Don't let depression isolate you from those who can help. Talk to your physician or a licensed mental health professional. As always, keep your physician informed of all medications and other treatments.

If you've been recently diagnosed with fibromyalgia and became depressed afterward, you may need time to grieve. After all, you've just been told you have a disorder with no known cure that may alter your life indefinitely. You will no doubt experience this as a major loss, and as with other losses, you need time to grieve. Grief is a natural way of dealing with loss and has five stages: *denial and isolation, anger, bargaining, depression,* and finally, *acceptance.* It takes time to move through these different stages, but seek help if you find yourself stalled at one stage or another. Acknowledge your feelings at each stage and then move on.

EMOTIONAL SUPPORT

Healthy people tend to develop support networks of friends and family upon whom they can rely in a rare crisis. Fibromyalgia sufferers need stronger support systems—ones they can count on night and day. A good rule of thumb is to have at least five family members and/or friends whom you can call on to help you. If you don't have five supporters at the ready, go get them! Don't wait for support to magically find you. Take the steps necessary to develop and nurture supportive relationships.

Remember the Golden Rule of relationships: If you want a friend, *you have to be a friend.* Breathe new life into old relationships by reaching out and offering your friendship. And make the effort to build relationships with new people.

Finding supportive people is easier than you might think. A great place to start is with a support group for people with fibromyalgia. These people will understand what you are going through on a very personal level. You won't have to describe your symptoms in detail; they will know what you mean and can empathize with your pain and suffering.

Don't allow support group meetings to turn into nonstop gripe sessions. Vent when you need to, then get back to more positive talk. If you notice a member constantly complaining and venting negative feelings, try to turn the conversation around to something more encouraging, like new research you've heard about or helpful ideas for goal-setting.

Support groups offer the latest news about fibromyalgia treatment and research on a regular basis, often in the form of a newsletter that contains invaluable information, tips, suggestions, and strategies. Such newsletters are generally loaded with practical ideas because the suggestions are contributed by those struggling with the disorder.

To find a support group in your area, contact the American Fibromyalgia Syndrome Association (for information on how to contact this association and others, check the resource listing at the back of this book). If you are a computer buff, there are many Web sites devoted to this issue. Tap into some of them and you'll generally find useful links to other sites. Bookmark your favorite Internet resources for easy reference.

If there is no local chapter or support group, you may want to consider starting one. If so, contact the organization's headquarters and tell them what you'd like to do. Many of these associations have booklets explaining how to create support groups, and they will be more than happy to provide tips on how to build a membership and how to prevent meetings from becoming too negative.

FAMILY MATTERS

Everyone needs and deserves love and support. When you have a chronic illness, you need it more than ever, and you turn to family members and close friends. Unlike the members of your health care team, your family and your friends don't make a cent when they assist you; they do it out of love. But even the most giving kind of love can wear thin if it feels like the relationship is a one-way street. Try to shift the focus away from yourself. Strive for balance, and look for ways to nourish and support the most important people in your life.

Ask for help, but don't overwhelm your loved ones with demands they can't meet. You have an ongoing, perhaps lifelong, condition. Spread out your requests for support among several people. Introduce yourself to other fibromyalgia patients at support group meetings, cultivate their friendship, and maintain contact with them.

If you're the super caretaker type who rarely complains, now is the time to speak up! Ask for help. Cry on a shoulder or two. Let others learn to take care of themselves a bit more. Stop trying to be a hero. You may be surprised to discover that the people in your life will love and accept you anyway.

If you have children, be considerate of their feelings and tell them what's going on. Tailor your explanations to your children's ages, and don't expect them to respond to your disorder like "little adults." Keep them informed about your condition and educate them about fibromyalgia, but don't overeducate them. Too much detail can confuse younger children and frighten older ones.

In Sickness and In Health

Chronic illness can place tremendous stress on a marriage or long-term relationship. This relationship is your cornerstone, so protect it. If you think it's a problem area, consider counseling immediately. As your symptoms worsen, or during flares, the stress on your partner is undeniable. He or she may feel helpless to ease your pain or angry at you for being sick. You may feel inadequate or guilty for not being the person you wish you could be. Or you may feel angry and hurt that your mate isn't more sensitive and understanding. Whatever the situation, the sooner you get help, the better.

Encourage your partner to become better informed about your disorder and allow him or her to vent deeply held feelings. If your partner knows that you're living with constant pain (even though you look "fine"), that you may experience flares (sometimes without warning), and that there will be times when your symptoms force a change in plans, then situations may be more easily accepted.

When your partner talks, learn to listen actively, past the actual words, to what he or she is really saying.

When you stop a moment to consider what it feels like to be in your partner's shoes, you'll be better able to appreciate how much your partner really loves you, despite frustrations, fear, or anger.

MAKE LOVE? ARE YOU KIDDING?

Very possibly the last thing on your mind these days is sex. You've had to redefine your life in every other aspect, and just the act of rethinking, adapting, and accepting the various aspects of your life with fibromyalgia can require enormous energy. When it comes to physical intimacy, my guess is you're probably exhausted and often just "not in the mood."

But before you write off sex as one more casualty of chronic illness, consider this: From a physiological point of view, one of the best stress reducers for both body and mind is sexual climax. Sex improves circulation, releases tension, and temporarily increases endorphin levels in the brain (which relieve pain and help us feel good). And physical intimacy can be an important component of emotional intimacy.

If your symptoms are so severe that even the slightest touch is too painful and the mere thought of a hug is intolerable, don't give up. Talk about it and search for ways to make intimacy work for you. Many people aren't comfortable talking about sex, even with their partners. But avoiding the topic isn't going to improve your situation. You're likely to discover your partner also needs to express his or her needs and feelings. Consider consulting a physical therapist or a gynecologist (if you are a woman). These experts may be able to guide you in choosing times and techniques that will work for you.

Be realistic and don't compare yourself to what you think is "normal." Our culture would have us believe we're abnormal if we don't engage in wild sex several times a day, but the fact is most people don't have that kind of libido. Sexual drive varies from person to person. Libido can be affected by anxiety, medications, depression, and many other physical and emotional factors. In addition, chronic illness can drain you of energy.

There are countless ways to show affection, but don't use your diagnosis as a reason to avoid physical intimacy. Dr. Connie O'Reilly, a clinical psychologist interested in the issue of sexual desire in people with fibromyalgia, makes these suggestions:

- **Address unresolved power struggles in your relationship.** When we feel powerless, we will do whatever we can to gain some of that control back, including being passive and withholding. Withholding your sexuality is a powerful way to express anger without having to confront issues directly. What ultimately happens, however, is that the underlying issues are never resolved and your partner is left feeling confused and resentful. Deal with power issues directly and openly. Get outside help to guide you through these struggles.
- **Pay attention to pain.** Pain during sex is not desirable and shouldn't be accepted. There are many

possible causes, so don't just assume it's a side effect of medication. Often the solution is simple, like changing positions or using lubrication.

- **Talk to your partner.** Convey your feelings and desires with honesty and candor. Even if your relationship is decades old, don't assume that you don't need to talk. Your partner cannot read your mind. On the flip side, be a good listener. Hear what your partner is trying to say.

- **Put sex on your "To Do" list.** I'm exaggerating, of course, but do consciously plan time to be close. If you use medications to control pain, timing may be especially important.

- **Pamper yourself.** Many people feel sexier when they feel attractive. Add essential oils to bath water and massages, wear clothes that make you feel good, and eat pleasurable, nutritious food. Try introducing massage into your intimacy time. Exercise and gentle stretches can increase your stamina and strength.

- **Creativity is key.** You don't need to swing from the chandeliers to have great sex. In fact, you don't even need sexual intercourse. Touching and cuddling can do wonders.

There are hundreds of self-help books on the market that deal with issues of intimacy and sexuality. I also suggest contacting the Arthritis Foundation (included in the list of resources at the back of this book) to request the booklet entitled "Living and Loving." It's filled with helpful ideas and suggestions.

TO WORK OR NOT TO WORK?

For many of us, this is not even a question—somebody's got to put bread on the table and that usually means outside employment, whether or not we feel up to it. Recent statistics reveal that approximately 90 percent of fibromyalgia patients who want to work are able to do so.

Sounds good, doesn't it? But these statistics don't reveal what the person with fibromyalgia goes through on the job. Another recent survey shows that 30 percent of these patients had to modify their job in some way to accommodate their condition, and another 30 percent had to change jobs, usually because of pain. Other factors include fatigue, cognitive difficulties, stress, and unsuitable work environments.

MAKING WORK EASIER

Holding down a job can increase your feelings of control and empowerment, but it can also add stress to your life. Only you can decide what's best for you. If you decide to keep working, here are some suggestions to make your worklife easier:

- Break down large or multifaceted jobs into smaller, more manageable pieces you can handle one at a time.

- When possible, adapt equipment to ease muscle strain. Try a phone rest or a speaker phone. Check the height of your desk, and use a comfortable and supportive chair. To test proper seat height, slip your hand under your hamstrings while sitting. If your hand doesn't fit, you need a footrest.
- Plan your day's activities so you don't need to walk a lot. Conversely, do not sit in one position for too long. Every 20 to 30 minutes, get up and stretch to reduce numbness and muscle strain.
- Avoid sitting near air conditioning vents.
- When you talk to someone, turn your chair to face him or her so you don't have to twist your body.
- Think about where you place frequently used items at your workstation. Arrange your desk so that you don't need to squat or stretch to reach your tools.
- Don't take work home. You've done enough.
- Accept the fact that you can't change your coworkers or employer. *You* are the one who must adapt.

If you work with a computer:

- Keep your wrists straight.
- Don't stretch your fingers to get at those faraway keys; move your arms.
- When typing, relax your thumbs and keep your fingers curved.
- Occasionally drop your arms to your sides and shake your fingers.

- Hold the mouse loosely.
- Use your whole arm to move the mouse, not just your hand.
- Sit as far from the monitor as you can. Use big fonts so you can move back.
- Take breaks often. Go outside, if possible.

YOUR RIGHTS IN SCHOOL AND AT WORK

The Americans with Disabilities Act requires publicly funded schools and businesses with more than 15 employees to accommodate people with disabilities, *including chronic illnesses.* You have a right to ask for adaptations that will help you work more comfortably. You may be eligible for medical treatment, disability pay, or job retraining through the workers' compensation system. Because this system is often abused, people who have genuine needs may have a difficult time getting coverage. Work with your primary care physician. You may need to write a two- to three-page report that cites the specifics about your condition, and attach your complete medical records. You could also be eligible for Social Security disability benefits (ranging from $350 to $1,000 monthly). To find out, call the Social Security Administration at 800-772-1213.

TAKE THIS JOB AND . . .

Before deciding to quit your job, ask yourself:

- What do I like best and least about my job?
- Am I satisfied with the work I currently do?
- Is this job good for my health?

- Is it possible to cut down my hours in my current job?
- What other jobs have I done and enjoyed?
- What skills do I have? What are my hobbies or interests? Could I turn any of these into a profitable business?
- If I change jobs, do I need to return to school?

Your occupational therapist can help you evaluate your options. He or she knows your physical limitations and abilities, as well as what jobs are available to you. Together you can come up with a plan.

SELF-EMPLOYMENT

For many reasons, more and more people today are self-employed, work at home, or telecommute. There are many advantages to self-employment, and most people who have made the change say they'd never go back to working for someone else. But telecommuting is not for everyone.

One of the biggest pluses of working at home is the chance to set your own hours. This means that during periods of flare, you don't need to worry about making it into the office. Perhaps your current employer is open to a work-at-home arrangement with you. This will certainly depend on the kind of work you do, the level of your position, if you are responsible for other people, and so on. Leaving a steady job to start your own business requires an enormous "leap of faith." If you are considering this option, you must ask yourself some important questions:

- Do I have a skill that can generate sufficient income?
- Do I have the discipline required to run a home-based business?
- Do I have the education, experience, and knowledge to handle every aspect of running a business? (If not, could I hire a bookkeeper, accountant, etc.?)
- Could I create public and private "zones" and leave my work behind me at the end of the day?
- Do I have the space I need to work at home?

Your local library has many resources on starting a home-based business and identifying those businesses that work best under these conditions. If you're considering this step, do some careful research to minimize the risks.

LOOK FOR (AND FIND) THE GOOD

Everything in life contains both good and bad elements. No matter what your situation, if you can find the good, you'll find your peace. Getting the most from life often involves an attitude change. Practice seeing the glass as half-full, rather than half-empty.

Many of our stress responses begin in our own imagination. Has a friend not returned your call because she's angry, or (more likely) because other events are keeping her occupied? Don't allow a vivid negative imagination to ruin your life. When you feel a stress reaction coming on, get in the habit of running a "reality check." Ask yourself, "Is it really important that another car beat me to that parking space?" Most of the things we let bother us are trivial. Save your concern for the things that really matter.

When you feel sorry for yourself, it can help to refocus on someone or something outside yourself. Look for ways to help others. In addition to providing a welcome distraction, being of service to someone else can provide a new, beneficial perspective on life.

For more ideas on how to enjoy life to the fullest, check the list of "100 Ways to Feel Better Right Now" in Chapter 13.

7

Getting the Most from Complementary/Alternative Medicine

If you've been diagnosed with fibromyalgia, odds are you already know the bad news: There's no known way to prevent the disorder or cure it. Coping with this condition day in and day out, year after year, can be relentlessly challenging. Recurrent, often constant muscle pain, headaches, fatigue, sleeplessness, and depression—and the frustrating search for a correct diagnosis and appropriate medical treatment—can wear down your body, tax your relationships, and leave you feeling much older than your years, both mentally and physically.

There is some good news, however. The debilitating range of fibromyalgia symptoms—from chronic muscle pain and severe fatigue to headaches and depression—*can* be controlled. You *can* recapture the life you may have lost. It *can* be done. But it will take persistence, patience, and the power of information.

Just as fibromyalgia is a collection of symptoms that can be caused by many different mechanisms or diagnoses, it is unlikely that any single therapy or treatment—whether conventional or nontraditional—will bring you the deep, long-term relief you seek. In fact, relying on one therapy alone almost guarantees failure. In my experience, people who cope well with fibromyalgia generally rely on an approach that integrates the best in traditional medical practice with sound nutrition and a variety of approaches drawn from the world of complementary and alternative medicine. Such a strategy can, in many cases, offer quick (if not immediate) symptom relief and can help minimize flare-ups.

Because the symptoms of fibromyalgia are so extensive and wide ranging, no single approach helps all of the people all of the time. In fact, what worked for you last year or last month may not do the trick today. Take some time to learn about your various options, explore several, and keep track of what works best for you, under what circumstances, and when.

THE GROWING DEMAND FOR COMPLEMENTARY/ALTERNATIVE MEDICINE

Ten years ago you had to search for tiny health food stores or obscure specialty shops to find a simple herbal tea. Today, extracts of St. John's wort, echinacea, and hundreds of other herbs and natural remedies line the shelves of Wal-Mart, K-Mart, CVS, and many other big chain stores across America. Mainstream supermarkets now carry soy milk, herbal teas, and a good selection of organic products. Even 7-Eleven sells convenient one-shot bottles of ginseng and travel packs of homeopathic medicines.

Dissatisfied with conventional medicine's focus on illness rather than wellness, consumers have been voting with their pocketbooks. Mainstream businesses have responded to the shift in demand. For the most part, mainstream medicine has lagged behind and done its best to ignore the growing public interest in "alternative" health care. But now, as consumer demand continues to swell, even conservative medical institutions like the American Medical Association and the National Institutes of Health have had to respond to the changing tide.

Unlike conventional medicine, with its focus on diagnosing and treating disease and suppressing symptoms, complementary/alternative medicine (CAM) is more likely to look at the entire person—body, mind, and spirit. In addition to treating immediate physical symptoms (like a runny nose or an aching back), these therapies typically take a more "holistic" approach to health and healing. CAM practitioners consider the underlying functioning of complex body systems (like the immune system), as well as the larger context of the patient's beliefs, personal circumstances, lifestyle choices, and external environment.

Complementary/alternative practitioners usually rely on gentler, less invasive diagnostic and therapeutic interventions than those routinely implemented by conventional physicians—often with fewer side effects. And most importantly, CAM approaches may provide relief (and occasionally even cures) when Western medicine falls short.

But that doesn't mean that all alternative therapies are right for all people. Some carry significant risks. Anything that is effective also has the potential to be dangerous when used improperly. Anyone considering using nontraditional approaches to help manage their fibromyalgia must take charge of their health by learning as much as possible about the various appropriate options before pursuing any treatment.

HOW DID IT ALL BEGIN?

With all the media coverage of late, it may seem as though the complementary/alternative medicine phenomenon is relatively new. Actually, much of what we think of today as nontraditional medicine is as traditional as it gets. Herbal therapies, Ayurvedic medicine, traditional Chinese medicine, and massage have been used to promote health and healing for thousands of years. It's really Western medicine (also known as *allopathic* medicine) that's the new kid on the block.

Much of our current national interest in CAM was sparked in 1971 during President Richard Nixon's historic trip to China. During the visit, *New York Times* reporter James Reston, suddenly stricken with acute appendicitis, underwent emergency surgery at the Anti-Imperialist Hospital in Beijing. Reston later wrote about his unexpected encounter with Eastern medicine, including how the strange Chinese practice of placing tiny needles in the skin relieved his postoperative pain *without medication*. Reston's fascinating reports brought the ancient healing practice of acupuncture to the attention of increasingly health-conscious Westerners.

At about the same time we were opening our minds to acupuncture, a growing number of Americans were tuning into transcendental meditation, or "TM," introduced by Maharishi Mahesh Yogi, personal guru to the Beatles. Those who practiced TM for relaxation and enlightenment began to discover its many health benefits, including its ability to lower blood pressure and ease chronic pain.

In the years to come, other unconventional therapies captured our attention. Some were championed by various physicians-turned-talk-show-guests/authors, including Bernie Siegel, Andrew Weil, Deepak Chopra, Dean Ornish, Christiane Northrup, and others. The sale of nutritional supplements grew steadily into a booming business. And more and more herbalists, acupuncturists, naturopaths, chiropractors, nutritionists, massage therapists, and yoga teachers set up shop across America.

In time, even the federal government had to officially recognize the growing groundswell of public interest in so-called alternative therapies. In 1992, the United States Congress set aside $2 million to establish the Office of Alternative Medicine (OAM) as part of the National Institutes of Health (NIH). Renamed the National Center for Complementary and Alternative Medicine (NCCAM) in 1998, the office disperses its now $68 million annual budget to fund research through nine specialty research centers around the country. These universities and medical centers are charged with investigating CAM's potential application in addiction, aging, arthritis, cardiovascular disease, craniofacial disorders, neurological conditions, and pediatrics.

WHERE IS IT ALL LEADING?

In one sense, the NIH is playing a game of catch-up. More and more Americans have already decided that their conventional M.D.s—those godlike healers (some physicians seem to think M.D. stands for minor deity) in whom they once put all their trust—no longer have all the answers when it comes to wellness, disease prevention, and effective treatment of chronic disorders. Many people have come to feel that their conventional doctors don't even ask the right questions.

In 1993, Harvard University researcher Dr. David Eisenberg reported in the *New England Journal of Medicine* the results of a 1990 survey revealing that as many as one in three Americans was using at least one form of unconventional therapy. The following year a Gallup Poll determined that 17 percent of Americans were using herbal supplements, a jump of 14 percent from the previous year.

Dr. Eisenberg subsequently reported in a 1998 issue of the *Journal of the American Medical Association* the results of a 1997 follow-up survey that showed that seven years later, 42 percent of Americans were using some form of unconventional therapy—a 25 percent increase since the first survey. During that same seven-year period, the use of herbal supplements jumped a noteworthy 380 percent, making herbal products the fastest growing segment of the CAM industry.

The most interesting (and most frightening) finding of both surveys was that most patients who use CAM therapies don't tell their medical doctors about it, perhaps fearing confrontation or ridicule. In fact, based on Eisenberg's second survey, more than 15 million adults in the United States routinely put themselves at risk for potentially dangerous interactions between their prescription medications and their "secret" CAM supplements.

As public interest in alternative and complementary practices has grown, the bastions of conventional Western medicine—medical schools and mainstream health care organizations—have begun to incorporate complementary medicine into their own programs and services. In 1993, New York City's Columbia University College of Physicians and Surgeons became one of the first medical schools in the country to begin exploring alternative therapies. Today the university's Richard and Hinda Rosenthal Center for Complementary and Alternative Medicine is one of NIH's CAM specialty centers and supports a number of projects—from studying the application of complementary/alternative medicine in women's health, to the relationship between religious beliefs and healing, to the development of electives in complementary medicine for the college's medical students. At the beginning of the millennium, two-thirds of all United States medical schools were offering electives in nontraditional therapies.

Big-city medical centers can no longer afford to ignore the trend and are scrambling to establish CAM clinics to meet the public's demand for access to qualified practitioners. At the Center for Integrative Medicine at Thomas Jefferson University Hospital in Philadelphia, board-certified physicians will not only check your heart and blood pressure, they'll also suggest treatment options that might include yoga, massage therapy, or acupuncture.

In Colorado, numerous integrative medicine programs combine traditional and nontraditional therapies. Many of these programs are affiliated with hospitals. I've taken part in this changeover. In addition to taking an integrative or collaborative approach in my own clinical practice, I have served as the medical director of alternative and complementary medicine for Centura Health—Colorado's largest network of medical offices, hospitals, and skilled nursing facilities. Centura realized that with 40 percent of the population using CAM therapies, the local medical establishment had an ethical and moral obligation to get involved, to help provide credible information, and to do our best to make sure that complementary medicine was practiced in a safe, rational way. Recently, I've had the privilege of working with Catholic Health Initiatives (CHI), a national organization based in Denver, to help guide and support efforts to establish integrative medicine programs at interested facilities across the country.

Even the American Medical Association (AMA) and its affiliate state and local medical societies can no longer ignore the trend. While not specifically endorsing complementary medicine, these organizations are encouraging their members to become more familiar with CAM modalities in order to more effectively discuss the proper use of these approaches with their patients.

Perhaps the most telling evidence of the popularity and effectiveness of certain alternative therapies is the fact that more and more health insurance companies now offer coverage for certain treatments—most commonly chiropractic and acupuncture. American Western Life of Foster City, California, was one of the first insurers to cover a wide range of complementary interventions. Oxford Health Plans—a managed care company serving 1.6 million members in New York, New Jersey, and Connecticut—was the first large medical insurer to offer its members a network of credentialed alternative care providers. A 1997 survey of Oxford subscribers showed that 75 percent were interested in adding alternative medical treatments and services to their current plan and that 33 percent had used alternative medicine in the past three years.

DOES CAM REALLY WORK?

Although most complementary practitioners argue that Western medicine has its drawbacks—pointing, for example, to drug side effects or new antibiotic-resistant strains of infection—the vast majority readily concede that Western medicine is absolutely peerless when it comes to acute and emergency care. Emergency situations call for emergency interventions. If you have a broken leg, you don't want an herb; you need a cast.

Conventionally trained health care practitioners have not been quick to return the compliment. More often than not, physicians turn a deaf ear when alternative practitioners and their satisfied clients suggest that their CAM therapies may be as effective as, or even better than, conventional medicine for promoting wellness, relieving chronic pain, and managing long-term illnesses.

It's not hard to understand why. Years of rigorous academic training makes skeptics out of the vast majority of conventional doctors and systematically instills in them an appetite for that "gold standard" of medical proof, the double-blind–placebo-controlled (DBPC) study.

The drawback in a strict adherence to the DBPC standard is that even Western medicine cannot meet it all the time. By most estimates, more than half of all conventional medical treatments have *not* been proven in DBPC research. Yet most conventional Western physicians continue to insist that CAM therapies are worthless unless they pass this test. This is clearly a double standard. If, in fact, Western medicine were restricted to only those therapies *proven* effective in DBPC studies, we doctors would have much less to offer our patients. The truth is that some therapies are very difficult, if not impossible, to study within this methodology.

The fact that academicians struggle with this challenge does not negate the practical value of the therapies in question. In other words, *a lack of research does not mean a lack of results*. And that's what patients care about—results. Patients are inclined to accept what seems to work rather than worry about academic hair-splitting.

Complementary therapies that have proven their clinical effectiveness for hundreds, even thousands, of years may not fit the conventional research protocols. But a growing number of studies do meet the most stringent scientific criteria and demonstrate conclusively the benefits of complementary or alternative interventions in well-defined situations.

For example, a 1997 panel organized by the National Institutes of Health concluded, after reviewing the scientific literature, that acupuncture can quell the nausea and vomiting associated with surgery, chemotherapy, and postoperative dental pain. The panel also identified a number of pain-related conditions for which acupuncture can work in combination with, or as an acceptable alternative to, standard treatments. These disorders include addiction, stroke, headache, menstrual cramps, tennis elbow, lower back pain, carpal tunnel syndrome, asthma, and fibromyalgia.

In 1998, the *Journal of the American Medical Association* presented the results of six scientific studies in its special issue on alternative medicine. Among the findings:

- Moxibustion (the burning of herbs to stimulate specific acupuncture points) is a safe, effective way to turn fetuses in a breech position.
- Chinese herbal medicine can be useful in treating irritable bowel syndrome.

- Yoga can help ease the pain of carpal tunnel syndrome.

Still missing in many of these studies is a theory or mechanism that explains the outcome in the scientific terms that conventionally trained physicians understand. That's why a certain percentage of physicians continue to categorize the whole field as irrelevant, believing that the public's interest in other healing systems will go the way of the pet rock.

But with over 40 percent of Americans now using complementary approaches, that may prove to be a shortsighted, even dangerous, position. If your conventional medical doctor falls into this category, you may want to consider shopping around for a more open-minded physician.

Hopefully, the health care delivery system of the future will integrate the scientific and technological strengths of Western medicine with the centuries-old body–mind–spirit orientation of complementary practice to provide each of us, in sickness and in health, the best of both worlds.

THE SIX BRANCHES OF CAM

With complementary/alternative practices, you will find more than three hundred therapies or modalities and hundreds more offshoots and variants. CAM approaches to health literally run the gamut from A to Z—from acupuncture to zone therapy. To make sense of this vast landscape, it's helpful to group similar therapies into broader categories. There are many ways to do this, and no one classification scheme is entirely complete or authoritative.

I prefer to classify CAM therapies on the basis of the mechanism(s) by which they work, or claim to work. I find that such a system is useful for both diagnosis and treatment. The disadvantage of this classification model is that some important systems of healing (for example, naturopathy, Ayurveda, and traditional Chinese medicine) involve multiple, complex mechanisms and therefore must be listed under several categories.

Using this system, the complementary/alternative modalities can be grouped into six broad categories:

> **Biochemical Therapies**—including general nutri-tion (diet, vitamins, and minerals), herbal medicine, Ayurveda, traditional Chinese medicine (TCM), chelation, and naturopathy. The effect of these therapies can be explained on the basis of what they do to the biochemistry of the body.

> **Structural Therapies**—including osteopathic manipulation, chiropractic, craniosacral therapy, naprapathy, kinesiology, physical therapy, massage, Rolfing, reflexology, and naturopathy. The effect of these interventions can be explained on the basis of what they do to the anatomic structures of the body.

> **Movement Functional Therapies**—including exercise, Alexander technique, Feldenkrais

method, Trager, *tai chi*, and yoga. The effect of these therapies can be attributed mostly to dynamic movement.

Energy Therapies—including TCM (acupuncture and acupressure), Ayurveda, yoga, Reiki, therapeutic touch, polarity therapy, biomagnetic therapy, some forms of osteopathic manipulation, some forms of chiropractic manipulation, craniosacral therapy, reflexology, homeopathy, and perhaps aromatherapy. These therapies are thought to work by correcting energy imbalances in the body.

Mind–Body Therapies—including psychological counseling, guided imagery, pet therapy, biofeedback, hypnosis, laughter therapy, prayer, meditation, Ayurveda, aromatherapy, and naturopathy. The effect of these therapies is generally attributed to changes in mind–body physiology.

Environmental Approaches—includes the avoidance of allergens, irritants, toxic substances, food additives, implants, and structures, and the correction of dysbiosis (microbial imbalances). These therapies all deal with the delicate balance that exists between one's body and the environment.

In the next five chapters we will be describing these therapies in detail and will examine what each can offer you in terms of managing your fibromyalgia symptoms and the side effects you may be experiencing with conventional medications.

As you know, general nutrition and herbal therapies—essentially biochemical approaches that offer many wellness strategies and programs to help you deal with common symptoms—were covered in great detail in Chapter 5. However, as you read further along, you will see that nutrition and herbal therapy also play key roles in naturopathy and in two alternative systems of healing, Ayurveda and traditional Chinese medicine. We'll be taking a close look at these approaches in Chapter 9.

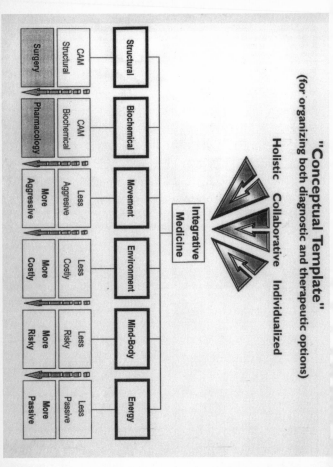

"Conceptual Template"
(for organizing both diagnostic and therapeutic options)

Holistic   Collaborative   Individualized

. . .

There are many possible ways to classify the more than 300 complementary and alternative therapies. For purposes of understanding what's available and when it's appropriate to use a given therapy, I believe the most useful method of classification is based on the presumed mechanism(s) of action. Using this scheme, it becomes apparent that the structural therapies are most appropriate for structural problems, the biochemical therapies are most appropriate for biochemical problems, and so on. The system therefore also becomes a way of diagnosing, from a holistic perspective, what imbalances are causing problems for a particular patient. The health care provider might ask, for example, are there anatomic /structural problems, biochemical imbalances, functional /movement problems, environmental issues, mind–body concerns, or energetic imbalances?

Most classification schemes used for complementary and alternative medicine (CAM) exclude conventional Western medicine and take the position that integrative medicine is the combination of Western medicine plus CAM. The problem with this approach is that it still implies a distinction between "us" and "them," a separation and tension between "this" and "that."

In reality, Western medicine fits very nicely in a classification scheme based on mechanisms of action. When you categorize all therapies on this basis, it becomes obvious that there is a hierarchy of more aggressive and less aggressive therapies in each therapeutic (and diagnostic) category. Doing surgery is clearly an anatomic/structural intervention; it just happens to be the most aggressive therapy in the structural category. Prescribing a medication (pharmacology) is clearly a biochemical intervention; it just happens to be the most aggressive therapy in the biochemical category. The Western medical therapies, in general, tend to be more aggressive, more costly, more risky, and more passive. The complementary therapies, in general, tend to be less aggressive, less costly, less risky, and less passive (meaning the patient is more actively involved).

The beauty of integrative medicine is that it neither forces aggressive therapies on patients when they are not needed, nor withholds aggressive interventions when they are needed. The most important first step is a thorough assessment and triage of the patient. If there is an urgent or emergency situation, go straight to Western medicine. If the situation is more chronic and poses no immediate threat, then it is worth trying less aggressive CAM interventions first and monitoring the outcomes closely. If the therapy you've chosen does not produce the desired results and the clinical situation is worsening or not improving, then it is totally appropriate to resort to more aggressive strategies.

GENERAL CAVEATS

As you delve into the world of complementary and alternative medicine, keep in mind that a good deal of what we know about CAM "best practices" is based on observational or anecdotal evidence. That means many interventions have not yet been investigated or proven in rigorous scientific studies. Also keep in mind that, in many cases, the long-term effects of various complementary therapies have not been determined.

While these caveats may hinder some physicians from recommending nontraditional approaches, growing numbers of fibromyalgia patients, less interested in academic debates, are finding the relief they're looking for by exploring and experiencing firsthand what CAM has to offer.

Remember, as with Western medical treatments, CAM therapies are not equally effective for all people in every circumstance. In fact, sometimes treatments may actually make things worse. For example, some forms of massage that are soothing to some patients can cause a flare-up of painful muscular aches and spasms in others. Therefore, it's particularly important to take the time to locate CAM practitioners with extensive experience in treating fibromyalgia in all its manifestations.

FOR HEALTH'S SAKE, KEEP THE COMMUNICATION CHANNELS OPEN

Be sure to discuss all potential CAM treatments and therapies with your conventional physician. Likewise, tell your complementary practitioners everything you're already doing on the conventional front.

This is not because you need anyone's permission to try a new approach, but because you want to do everything possible to cultivate *a team approach*. Each member of your health care team should be able to evaluate your total strategy and tell you whether any of the therapies you're considering are ill-advised. If any of your health care providers is not receptive to collaboration, you may wish to replace that person with someone willing to treat you within an integrative framework.

CHOOSING THE BEST COMPLEMENTARY PRACTITIONERS FOR YOU

The best practitioners are technically competent, have a balanced, collaborative philosophy, and conduct themselves in a professional manner. Here's what to look for:

TECHNICAL COMPETENCE

Certification/Licensure—Has the practitioner been accredited by a national or state body for this discipline, if applicable? You'll find a list of CAM accrediting organizations at the back of this book.

Institutional endorsement—Did the practitioner graduate at the top of his or her class or at the bottom?

Peer endorsement—Does this practitioner get good reviews from others in the health care field?

Patient endorsement—Is this practitioner praised by patients? Patients sing the praises of practitioners who get results. For some of the unregulated therapies, this may be your best indicator of competence.

Experience—Is this a "sideline" or the main focus of the practitioner's clinical practice? Ask how long he or she has been working in this specialty and discuss his or her experience and results with specific conditions. For example, some acupuncturists specialize in pain control, while others specialize in infertility or drug withdrawal.

BALANCED, COLLABORATIVE PHILOSOPHY

Team/Partnership approach—Does the practitioner feel comfortable working in partnership with the patient and with the medical community? If a practitioner says all Western medicine is "poison" or "evil," run, don't walk, in the opposite direction!

Communication—Does the practitioner feel comfortable talking with medical doctors or sending them consultation and/or progress notes regarding shared patients?

Recognition of limitations—Ask the practitioner what conditions he is comfortable treating and which he would refer to another practitioner. No single practitioner working in one discipline can successfully treat all conditions or patients. If he can't give you a clear answer, that's a red flag.

PROFESSIONALISM

Liability insurance—Does the practitioner carry liability insurance? It's a necessary part of responsible practice.

Projected number of treatments and cost—Is the practitioner able to give at least a rough estimate before you start treatment?

Projected time frame—How soon can you expect to experience some improvement? To avoid wasting time and money, you should know when to determine whether treatment has been successful or it's time to move on to a different approach.

RELIEF SYMPTOM-BY-SYMPTOM

To help guide you through the next five chapters, the following chart indicates some of the most common fibromyalgia symptoms and the corresponding complementary/alternative treatments that may provide some measure of relief.

FIBROMYALGIA	Chronically Painful Muscles	Severe Fatigue and Sleep Disorders	Circulatory Problems	Headaches	Premenstrual Syndrome	Upper Respiratory Infection	Digestive Problems	Depression
Acupressure	✓	✓	✓	✓	✓		✓	✓
Acupuncture	✓	✓	✓	✓	✓	✓	✓	✓
Aromatherapy	✓	✓	✓	✓	✓	✓	✓	✓
Ayurveda	✓	✓	✓	✓			✓	✓
Biofeedback	✓	✓	✓	✓				
Biomagnetic Therapy	✓	✓	✓	✓				
Chinese Herbal Medicine		✓	✓	✓			✓	
Chinese Medical Diet							✓	
Chiropractic	✓			✓	✓		✓	
Craniosacral Therapy	✓			✓				
Electrostatic Massage	✓		✓	✓				
Exercise	✓	✓						
Herbal/Dietary/Nutritional Therapies	✓	✓		✓	✓	✓	✓	✓
Homeopathy	✓	✓		✓	✓	✓	✓	✓

FIBROMYALGIA	Chronically Painful Muscles	Severe Fatigue and Sleep Disorders	Circulatory Problems	Headaches	Premenstrual Syndrome	Upper Respiratory Infection	Digestive Problems	Depression
Hydrotherapy	✓	✓	✓	✓		✓	✓	
Laughter Therapy	✓		✓					✓
Massage	✓	✓	✓	✓			✓	
Meditation		✓			✓			
Mind–Body Therapies	✓	✓	✓	✓			✓	✓
Movement Therapies	✓		✓	✓				✓
Naturopathy	✓	✓	✓	✓	✓	✓	✓	✓
Osteopathy			✓	✓				
Reflexology	✓	✓	✓	✓	✓		✓	✓
Reiki			✓					✓
Tai Chi/Qigong			✓					
Therapeutic Touch	✓		✓	✓			✓	
Trigger Point Myotherapy	✓		✓					
Ultrasound			✓					
Yoga	✓	✓	✓	✓	✓		✓	✓

8

Energy Therapies

TRADITIONAL CHINESE MEDICINE
ACUPUNCTURE, ACUPRESSURE, CHINESE HERBAL MEDICINE,
CHINESE DIETARY THERAPY

AYURVEDIC HEALING
HOMEOPATHY
BIOMAGNETIC THERAPY
ELECTROSTATIC MASSAGE
POLARITY THERAPY
REIKI
THERAPEUTIC TOUCH

The alternative and complementary approaches grouped under the umbrella term "energy therapies," in my opinion, hold the most potential for the future of medicine. They are also the ones that most directly challenge the prevailing Western biochemical model. For conventional doctors, the energy therapies are the most intellectually, academically, and professionally risky because they cannot be explained by prevailing dogma.

In simple terms, conventional Western medicine is based on a model consisting of anatomic structures and systems that are sustained by biochemical processes. Traditional Chinese medicine (TCM) and Ayurvedic healing are based on a completely different model—one based on the flow of energy within the body (called *chi* in TCM, *prana* in Ayurveda). In these healing traditions, illness is attributed to energetic imbalances, and health is restored when the imbalances are corrected.

From a conventional medical standpoint, all this is nonsense. Conventional physicians point to an absence of consistent anatomic structures that correspond with acupuncture points and meridians (energy pathways) of TCM. They also are likely to explain the clinically demonstrated effects of acupuncture, for example, in terms of the biochemistry of endorphin release.

Those who have taken the time to investigate the energy therapies know, however, that several studies have documented that our bodies have areas of low electrical resistance and high electrical conductivity—these correspond to the acupuncture points and meridians. This being the case, the concept of electrons (a current) following the paths of least resistance in the body becomes plausible, and the concept of *chi* or *prana* seems less farfetched.

Therapeutic touch, which paradoxically often involves no touching at all, is another type of energy therapy that has been tossed aside by skeptics. In fact, there are scores of well designed scientific studies documenting physiologic changes as a result of therapeutic touch, including accelerated wound healing, increased hemoglobin and oxygen levels, and even *in vitro* altered enzyme activity. Unfortunately, to date such studies have been published mostly in nursing journals or CAM journals. Despite the impeccable scientific rigor of some of these studies, they have usually been excluded from publication in mainstream medical journals.

That's because the biomedical model is clearly called into question once you acknowledge that one person can cause physiologic changes in another person without even touching them. Such controversy undoubtedly contributes to intellectual indigestion and fears of lost credibility in the typically conservative editorial boards that decide what is worthy of publication in medical journals.

Clearly the Western biomedical model is inadequate to explain many of the well documented responses to energetic interventions. Yet these are the therapies that are the most exciting to many integrative physicians because they have the greatest potential to challenge our thinking and expand our understanding of how the human body works.

In this chapter we'll be looking at a number of energy-based approaches that can offer some measure of relief to the person with fibromyalgia. These include traditional Chinese medicine (acupuncture, acupressure, Chinese herbal medicine, and Chinese dietary therapy), Ayurveda, homeopathy, biomagnetic therapy, electrostatic massage, polarity therapy, Reiki, and therapeutic touch.

TCM and Ayurveda straddle the energy-based category and the biochemical category, as medical professionals trained in the Western tradition often try to explain their effects in terms that are more familiar to conventional medicine.

Similarly, many practitioners of reflexology would group that modality with the energy therapies, maintaining that the overall goal of treatment is to facilitate a healthy balance and flow of bodily energy. You'll find information on reflexology in Chapter 10.

TRADITIONAL CHINESE MEDICINE

Traditional Chinese medicine (TCM) is one of the oldest healing systems in the world and has been practiced in China and Eastern Asia for nearly five thousand years. In the Eastern tradition, TCM is thought of as an energy therapy; in the West, the conventional medical community likes to explain the effects of TCM in terms of the biochemical model they already understand.

Two concepts are central to TCM: balance and flow. The TCM practitioner helps the individual achieve internal balance (*yin* and *yang*), as well as balance with the external environment. The second concept, flow, relates to the energy or life force (*chi*) circulating within each individual.

According to TCM, the nature of your illness depends on the particular imbalance between your *yin* and *yang*. Too much *yin*, for example, results in "cold" symptoms like chills; too much *yang* results in "hot" symptoms like fever. Different organs are characterized as *yin* or *yang*; the liver, for example, is *yin*, while the stomach is *yang*.

Chi is thought to move through the body along 12 energy pathways called *meridians*. Whether you call it *chi* (Eastern) or *electrons* (Western), correcting energy imbalances can have profound effects on physiology. Research has shown repeatedly that the acupuncture points and meridians are actually low-resistance electrical pathways, much like an electric grid for the body. TCM holds that when *chi* is blocked or out of balance, illness results. Studies have also shown that pathology (whether a fracture, a tumor, a cut, a muscle spasm, etc.) is accompanied by abnormal electrical activity, and that correcting the abnormal electrical activity can often bring improvement.

Chi can become weak, stagnant, or misdirected. Weakened *chi* can result in loss of appetite, dizzy spells, and a weak pulse. Stagnant or blocked *chi* can lead to tightness of the chest, abdominal pain, and painful and/or irregular periods. Misdirected *chi*, in which the energy flows in the wrong direction, can cause asthma, coughs, vomiting, and fainting. Re-establishing the normal flow of *chi* and balancing *yin* and *yang* is thought to restore health and prevent illness.

In traditional Chinese medicine, treatment may involve a combination of Chinese herbal medicine, acupuncture, acupressure, Chinese medical massage (*tui na*), exercise (such as *tai chi*), and dietary therapy. TCM differs from Western medicine in that it focuses on the entire body, not just the specific parts that are affected by disease or injury. When Western medicine finally embraces the inseparability of energy and physiology, we can expect to see dramatic changes in health care.

Attempts to translate TCM terminology into Western terms can sometimes be confusing. However, there are many studies documenting its clinical effectiveness for a wide variety of conditions including arthritis, asthma, cerebral palsy, colitis, depression, diabetes, drug withdrawal, hay fever, herpes, impotence, infertility, insomnia, menopause, nausea (associated with chemotherapy, pregnancy, or surgery), premenstrual syndrome, sciatica, stroke, and chronic pain.

ACUPUNCTURE

Acupuncture is an ancient technique that originated in China at least 2,500 years ago. The painless insertion of very fine disposable needles in points along the body's meridians is intended to relieve symptoms by correcting energy imbalances and restoring the normal, healthy flow of energy.

Many Western-trained physicians and researchers prefer a more scientific (biochemical) explanation and hold that acupuncture works by releasing the body's endorphins—peptides secreted in the brain that relieve pain and promote feelings of well-being.

The acupuncture points and meridians have repeatedly been shown to be low-resistance electrical pathways, and the use of acupuncture needles or acupressure changes the electron flow (current) along these pathways. If the Eastern terminology (*chi, yin* and *yang*) is intimidating or confusing, it may be easier to think in the Western, scientifically neutral terms of charge, electrons, electricity, and current which are devoid of cultural or metaphysical interpretations.

Regardless of whether you believe in energetic or biochemical mechanisms, acupuncture has proven useful for pain control, the nausea associated with chemotherapy or pregnancy, drug withdrawal (including nicotine withdrawal), stress reduction, and the management of gastrointestinal problems and menstrual disorders. When used alongside conventional medical treatment, it can also provide relief for patients suffering from osteoarthritis, asthma, and headaches. Many patients have had good results using acupuncture to treat the muscle pain, fatigue, and depression that are common in fibromyalgia.

Acupuncture has been effective in reducing the chronic pain associated with fibromyalgia in some patients. To treat back pain, for example, the practitioner will usually insert needles along the paraspinal muscles that straddle the spine, as well as in some points along the arms or legs. He may also work with specific tender points or trigger points that may be responsible for causing both localized and radiating pain.

Most acupuncturists working today use presterilized disposable needles that come packaged in sealed envelopes. The number of needles used, and their placement, varies from person to person, even from session to session, depending on the results being sought. Some practitioners swab the acupuncture point with alcohol before inserting the needles. Others may use a treatment called *moxibustion*. This consists of applying heat directly above acupuncture points by means of small bundles of smoldering herbs, usually mugwort leaf. Moxibustion frequently accompanies the insertion of needles, but it can be used alone.

Sometimes the needles are hooked up to tiny wires that deliver a very weak electrical current to the acu-points. In a study published in the *British Medical Journal*, one group of fibromyalgia patients was treated with electroacupuncture, and the other was treated with acupuncture needles that were inserted less deeply, at a distance from traditional acupuncture sites, and with a weaker electrical current. The patients who received the electroacupuncture reported less morning stiffness, less overall pain, and better quality of sleep.

Once the needles are inserted, you usually lie quietly for 30 to 60 minutes. The acupuncturist will then remove the needles and discard them. You may occasionally develop a slight bruise if the needle has hit a blood vessel, but that happens only rarely.

The number of treatments depends on your condition. Sometimes one or two visits can do the trick; other times six, eight, or 10 treatments might be in order. And once you feel that you're back on track, you may want to schedule treatment on a regular basis; many people opt for monthly or quarterly sessions to stay in balance.

Choose an acupuncturist or a physician who is certified by the National Certification Commission for Acupuncture and Oriental Medicine (NCCAOM). This organization publishes an annual directory of board-certified practitioners. You can also contact the American

Association of Oriental Medicine (AAOM) and request a list of qualified acupuncturists in your area.

Currently, medical doctors (M.D.s) and chiropractors can perform acupuncture in many states; some practitioners are excellent, some are not. To experience maximum benefit, it's important to seek out a qualified practitioner. In addition to good training, it takes years of ongoing practice to become a superior acupuncturist. You cannot expect this level of skill from someone who's taken a weekend course in acupuncture or who merely dabbles in it as a sideline. Be sure your practitioner has had substantial training and devotes a large share of his or her ongoing clinical practice to acupuncture.

CAUTION—If you have an infection or are prone to bleeding easily, check with your physician before undergoing acupuncture.

ACUPRESSURE

Acupressure, like acupuncture, is based on the concept of energy (*chi*) circulating through the body's pathways (meridians). When *chi* is flowing freely, you remain healthy and in harmony; when *chi* is stagnant, overstimulated, or unbalanced, you become ill.

One of the best known forms of acupressure is called *shiatsu*, a Japanese word meaning "finger pressure." Acupressure uses many of the same points as acupuncture, but the practitioner uses deep finger pressure instead of needles. The technique is particularly helpful for stress-related symptoms such as headaches, neck and back pain, depression, anxiety, and insomnia. Other conditions that respond well to treatment include nausea, motion sickness, constipation, allergies, menstrual problems, and muscle aches. Obviously, if you are bothered by tender point pain, acupressure is not a good choice.

If you're suffering from generalized pain and stiffness, especially in the shoulder and neck area, lie face down on a comfortable surface and have a partner place the pads of his thumbs on either side of your spine and apply gentle pressure by putting a little weight over the thumbs. Start at the top vertebra and work down the spine one vertebra at a time.

Acupressure can also be self-administered. Consult a practitioner or pick up a self-help guide to learn about the different acupoints. When you have identified the point that coincides with your symptom, press it lightly with one finger. Increase the pressure gradually until you're pressing as firmly as you can. Hold this pressure steadily until you feel a faint, even pulse at the point; this should take between three to 10 minutes, perhaps longer. (You may feel some discomfort; if the pressure is really painful, ease up.) Release the pressure slowly.

If trigger-point blockages are a problem for you, try tennis ball acupressure, another technique you can do on your own. Simply place a tennis ball between a trigger point and an immovable object, such as a wall or the floor. When you lean into the ball, you compress the trigger point, forcing out the fluids that have built up in that area.

When performing acupressure, concentrate on your breathing; deep breathing helps the pressure points release pain or tension and increases the flow of energy, blood, and lymphatic fluid throughout your body. For best results, wear comfortable clothing.

In addition to its healing benefits, acupressure may help you stay well. The release of muscle tension increases the flow of blood and nutrients to the tissues, promoting physical and emotional relaxation.

Unlike acupuncturists, acupressure therapists are not licensed. To find a trained specialist, contact the American Association of Oriental Medicine.

CAUTION—If you have a chronic condition or illness, check with your physician before trying acupressure. Don't try acupressure just before or after a heavy meal, while bathing, or within four hours of taking any drugs or medication, including alcohol. You can perform the procedure every day, but limit your sessions to an hour. Releasing too much energy can cause nausea or headache.

CHINESE HERBAL MEDICINE

Herbs have always played a central role in traditional Chinese medicine. TCM, in fact, recognizes more than 6,000 healing substances, grouped by four basic properties: hot, cold, warm, and cool. Herbalists choose plants that can help balance conditions that are caused by excessive heat or cold. A "hot" herb, such as cinnamon bark, may be prescribed for an "inner cold" condition, such as chronic diarrhea or cold hands and feet. A "cool" herb, such as chrysanthemum flower, can correct an "inner heat" condition, such as rapid onset inflammation involving headache and fever.

Herbs are also classified by the five flavors: pungent, sour, sweet, bitter, or salty. Each flavor influences a certain organ—pungent for the lungs, sour for the liver, sweet for the spleen or pancreas, bitter for the heart, and salty for the kidneys. In Chinese philosophy, the concept of organs is much broader than it is in the West. The Chinese "heart," for example, refers to the physical heart as well as clarity of mind.

Chinese herbs are generally prescribed in combinations of five to 10 at a time. They are usually prepared in a soup or a strong tea to be drunk at room temperature (never hot). Many herbs are also available in powder or pill form, as tinctures, and as pastes that can be applied to the skin. Be prepared to be patient. Like Western herbal remedies, Chinese herbal treatments take some time to work.

If you live in a city with a large Asian population, you should be able to find a TCM practitioner who was trained in China or Taiwan or at one of the programs accredited by the National Certification Commission for Acupuncture and Oriental Medicine (NCCAOM). If not, look for a medical doctor, osteopath, chiropractor, or licensed acupuncturist who has received at least 500 hours of training in Chinese herbalism and who routinely applies this knowledge in clinical practice. You want to avoid practitioners that have just taken a weekend course or who may have had good training but only dabble occasionally in this field. My recommendation is to find a practitioner who meets NCCAOM standards and who practices this speciality full-time.

CAUTION—To avoid potentially serious interactions, make sure you tell *all* of your health care practitioners about *all* prescriptions and herbs you are taking. Some Chinese herbs can be poisonous in large doses. In Western medicine we are often reminded that the only difference between a medicine and a poison is the dose. This is just as true with complementary therapies.

CHINESE DIETARY THERAPY

Chinese dietary therapy is considered a powerful tool and is used in conjunction with acupuncture and herbs. In fact, food and medicine are considered equally important. Foods are used to strengthen digestion, increase vitality, and balance the body's energy.

For a long, healthy life, traditional Chinese dietary therapy recommends bland, unprocessed foods. Natural foods—homegrown and chemical-free—are considered the best choices. Meat is generally limited to two to three ounces per meal, with red meat limited to about six ounces a week.

Foods are classified as warm, neutral, or cold. A person diagnosed with a "warm" condition works toward balance by eating "cooling" foods.

AYURVEDIC HEALING

Ayurveda—a Sanskrit word meaning "longevity knowledge"—is an ancient system of healing from India. Ayurvedic treatments all strive to create internal harmony and balance with diet, exercise, meditation, herbal therapy, and other therapies. Ayurvedic medicine has become increasingly popular in the United States in recent years, thanks to the best-selling books and television appearances of physician Deepak Chopra. Dr. Chopra was born and raised in India, studied and practiced Western medicine in the United States, and then managed to integrate powerful Ayurvedic therapies into his conventional medical practice.

At the root of Ayurvedic medicine is the holistic philosophy that each person has a vital energy, known as *prana*, found in various internal energy centers, called *chakras*. An imbalance of *prana* is thought to cause illness. This balance can be restored through a variety of interventions involving diet, yoga, lifestyle modifications, nutritional supplements, herbs, stress reduction techniques, meditation, and individualized therapies.

The Ayurvedic practitioner develops a personalized treatment plan for each patient by analyzing his or her constitutional makeup. According to Ayurvedic philosophy, each person contains a particular proportion of the universe's five elements—earth, air, fire, water, and ether (or space)—which combine to express the three *doshas* or basic constitutional types: *vata, pitta,* and *kapha*.

Vata, or wind, combines air and space. It is said to influence the movement of cells and fluid through the body and thoughts through the mind. People who are strongly influenced by *vata*, say Ayurvedic healers, are active and often restless.

Pitta, or bile, is made up of fire and regulates the body's metabolic activities. Those who are influenced by *pitta* may be competitive and aggressive.

The third dosha, *kapha,* or phlegm, is made up of earth and water and accounts for the body's physical strength, stability, and recuperative powers. A person whose makeup is predominantly *kapha* typically has a heavy, muscular body and a serene personality.

A person's natural makeup, called his *prakriti,* is a balance of the three *doshas.* Every *prakriti* contains elements of all the *doshas,* but only one predominates. Ayurvedic healers believe that if you live the life your *prakriti* dictates, you will remain in balance, in harmony, and in good health.

An Ayurvedic practitioner will closely examine your pulse, tongue, nails, eyes, face, and posture, and ask you detailed questions about your life. He or she will design an individualized health plan for you based on your physical examination and medical history, and will recommend a combination of herbs, nutrition, massage, yoga postures, breathing exercises, and meditation.

By taking into account the uniqueness of each individual and the mind, body, spirit, and energy factors that affect health, Ayurvedic medicine aims to treat the whole person. This approach can be quite helpful for people with stress-related conditions or chronic disorders.

THE AYURVEDIC DIET

Dietary recommendations are based on the seasons and on the particular elements of your *dosha.* Foods are classified on the basis of whether they increase (stimulate) or decrease (pacify) each *dosha.*

To pacify	Eat	Avoid
Vata	spices; heavy, warm, oily, moist foods; eat at regular meal times	raw, dry, cold, or frozen foods; leafy vegetables
Pitta	salads; cooling herbs and spices	alcohol; meat; sour, salty, spicy, and fried foods
Kapha	plenty of vegetables, salads; dry, light foods; spices	sweet and salty foods; dairy; fried foods; frozen foods

The qualities of any given food change with different preparation techniques, so you would include or exclude particular foods depending on how they're prepared. For example, if you were following a *vata*-pacifying diet, you would avoid dry oatmeal (served cold and dry as granola) but could eat cooked oatmeal, which is warm and moist. You would avoid cold fruit juice but could drink it warmed.

Other dietary rules apply to all of the *doshas* and concern food combinations. Cooked and raw foods are not eaten at the same meal. Fruits are eaten separately from other foods. Milk is not taken with yogurt. Milk and yogurt are not mixed with citrus, fish, meat, or eggs. Vegetarian diets are generally encouraged, usually a lacto-vegetarian diet (milk and cheese are permitted, but not meat, fish, chicken, or eggs).

The *doshas* are influenced by the environment, so your dietary prescription will change with the seasons of the year. It's important to consult a qualified practitioner for guidelines.

CAUTION—Ayurvedic healers are not currently required to be licensed or certified in the United States. If you're already taking prescription medicine, talk to your doctor before using any Ayurvedic herbs or medicines. Some may contain dangerous substances such as lead, mercury, and arsenic; avoid any that contain even the smallest amounts of these ingredients.

AYURVEDIC REMEDIES FOR PAIN RELIEF AND RESTFUL SLEEP

If you, like many people with fibromyalgia, find it difficult to sleep, a variety of Ayurvedic remedies may provide some relief:

- Ginger, capsaicin, and curcumin may be helpful in controlling pain and inflammation. See the section in Chapter 5 for more details on these herbal treatments.
- A cup of warm milk before going to bed can bring on more restful sleep. If you don't like plain milk, add a pinch of nutmeg; some blanched or crushed almonds, along with a pinch of nutmeg and a pinch of cardamom (the nuts can be prepared in a nut grinder or coffee grinder); or

try garlic milk, prepared with 1 c milk, ¼ c water, and 1 clove of fresh chopped garlic, boiled gently until 1 c of liquid remains.

- Tart cherries can help ease pain and therefore relieve the stress and mental fatigue that can keep you from resting comfortably. Eat 20 a day to help you sleep. This Ayurvedic remedy is supported by a study reported in the *Journal of Natural Products* (1999). Researchers at Michigan State University found that 20 tart cherries contained between 20 to 25 mg of a special class of bioflavonoids called anthocyanins known to be 10 times more effective than aspirin at relieving inflammation and reducing pain. Cherries are also a source of powerful antioxidants. Apples and pineapple have similar anti-inflammatory properties.

- A cup of tomato juice, with 2 teaspoons natural sugar and 2 pinches of nutmeg, drunk between 4:00 P.M. and 5:00 P.M., followed by dinner between 6:00 P.M. and 7:00 P.M., can also help bring on a sound sleep.

- Another Ayurvedic remedy that may help is an herbal mixture of 1 part tagar, 1 part valerian root powder, and 1 part chamomile. Take ¼ teaspoon of this powdered mix with a little warm water before going to bed.

- Chamomile tea, long used as a sleep aid in folk remedies around the world, may also help you get a good night's rest.

- A soothing warm oil massage before going to bed can be very relaxing and sleep inducing. Use sesame oil, brahmi oil, or jatamamsi oil, slightly warmed, and massage into the scalp and the soles of the feet.
- A warm bath or shower at bedtime will soothe *vata* and promote sleep.
- Yoga meditation is also effective.

HOMEOPATHY

Homeopathy, developed in Germany over two hundred and fifty years ago, uses highly diluted substances from plants, animals, and minerals as medicine. This healing system is based on the precept that "like cures like." While a conventional physician would tend to recommend a standard pharmaceutical remedy (such as acetaminophen) to reduce fever, a homeopathic practitioner would recommend a highly diluted remedy derived from a substance that actually causes fever in a healthy person. The diluted remedy is thought to stimulate the body's own protective healing response, somewhat like an immunization does.

Some homeopathic remedies are so diluted that if you tried to measure the concentration of active ingredient, you wouldn't find any! Thus many physicians reject homeopathy because it cannot be conventionally explained on a biochemical basis. Skeptical physicians attribute any benefit to the placebo response. In other words, they say, "It works because you expect it to work."

However, a number of double-blind–placebo-controlled studies have documented statistically significant responses to certain homeopathic remedies that cannot be explained by the placebo response. When confronted with this evidence, skeptical physicians still say, "I wouldn't believe it, even if it were true!"

At this time we can only speculate as to the mechanism of action at work in homeopathy, but it probably can be classified as one of the therapies that cause energy changes in the body. One clue supporting this theory is that the effect of homeopathic remedies can be neutralized by strong magnetic fields. In light of this, it's best not to use homeopathic remedies along with acupuncture or magnetic therapy.

Another tenet of homeopathy is that the patient is not his disease. In other words, not every treatment works on every patient, and each patient must be seen as an individual, not as an illness. This holistic philosophy is one of the pillars of alternative medicine.

USING HOMEOPATHIC REMEDIES

Homeopathic remedies should not be used as the only treatment for acute illness or medical emergencies. They are most effective when used to treat chronic conditions such as allergies, chronic fatigue syndrome, skin problems, headaches, premenstrual syndrome, colds and flu, and stress-related disorders. They are safe, however, to use with any medication you are taking, and can be taken by children, the elderly, and even pets.

There are about two hundred to three hundred commonly used homeopathic remedies, each designed to target a specific symptom. Preparations in tablet, powder, wafer, and liquid forms may be prescribed by a homeopathic physician or bought over the counter in health food stores, pharmacies, and grocery stores. Certain over-the-counter remedies are targeted to common ailments such as insomnia, colds, flu, sore throat, and headaches. For relatively minor, self-limited problems, you can use these preparations to treat yourself.

If you're using homeopathic remedies on your own, look for products with a potency in the range of 6c to 12c. The number preceding "c" indicates how many hundred times the remedy has been diluted. The most diluted forms are, paradoxically, thought to be the most potent. A professional homeopath may use products with potencies of 30c or higher, but it's best to start out on the lower end if you're doing it yourself.

If you're using a homeopathic remedy in tablet form, be careful not to touch the pills. Pour the tablets into the bottle cap, then tip them directly onto or under your tongue. If you spill any, throw them away. Don't take anything by mouth for 15 minutes before or after taking the tablets, especially mint, mint-flavored toothpaste, coffee, or tea.

Keep homeopathic remedies in their original container, away from heat, sunlight, and strong aromas (such as perfumes, camphor, and eucalyptus) which may cause contamination.

For chronic conditions, it's best to check with a professional homeopath who will take an extensive medical history and discuss your physical and psychological symptoms before prescribing a remedy tailored to your individual needs. Response times vary from minutes to months, and the remedies can work in conjunction with most other conventional and/or complementary therapies.

In one double-blind study reported in the *British Medical Journal*, 24 patients with fibromyalgia reported significant improvement after taking one of three homeopathic preparations that had been targeted to their specific symptoms:

- **Arnica 30c**—Appropriate in cases where the pain makes you feel bruised or beaten. If this remedy is useful, relief will be quite rapid, usually within 24 hours. Take every four or five hours, up to four or five doses in a day.
- **Bryonia 6c**—Can help people whose pain dictates that they remain completely immobile because motion intensifies the discomfort. Take three times daily for two days, then once a day for a week.
- **Rhus tox 30c**—A useful remedy for those whose pain is accompanied by anxiety and restlessness and who find that hot compresses and hot baths bring relief from pain and stiffness. Take three times daily for two days, then once a day for a week.

Licensing requirements for homeopathic practitioners can vary from state to state. Many homeopaths have professional training, such as a degree in medicine, osteopathy, or naturopathy.

CAUTION—Homeopathy is incompatible with other energy therapies and thus should not be used simultaneously. Consult a homeopathic practitioner before taking any of these medications on your own to treat a chronic disorder.

BIOMAGNETIC THERAPY

The use of magnets to restore or improve health has a long and somewhat checkered history. Some claim that Cleopatra used a magnetic lodestone to maintain her youthful appearance. In the late 1700s, mesmerism (an old term for hypnosis) came to be associated with the term "animal magnetism," casting an air of charlatanism on the medical use of magnets. This historical linkage to questionable therapies provided by unsavory individuals is still an obstacle for acceptance in the eyes of many clinicians.

More recently, however, a variety of respected researchers have published scientific studies on the use of biomagnets and pulsed electromagnetic fields (PEMF) in the treatment of a variety of conditions, including osteoarthritis, neurologic disorders, chronic pain, and psychiatric disorders.

Biomagnetic therapy appears to have two main effects on the body: improved blood flow and movement of charge/electrons caused by current induction. When a biomagnet (different from an ordinary refrigerator door magnet or an industrial magnet) is placed on a specific part of the body, blood flow through that area is increased. This improves the oxygen supply to cells, stimulates metabolism, and encourages the elimination of waste products from the area.

Thermography—a graphic demonstration of temperature changes within the body—shows that biomagnets can actually enhance blood flow on *both* sides of the body, not just where the magnet is placed. Such "nonlocal" effects defy Western medical explanation. The nonlocal effect of magnetic therapy is easier to explain in terms of the minute electric currents induced in the body by the magnetic fields. The induced currents follow the path of least resistance—which happens to be the acupuncture points and meridians.

Therefore, in a sense, magnetic therapy has effects similar to those of acupuncture because both modalities influence the flow of electricity in the body. In fact, magnets have been used effectively by some TCM practitioners over acupuncture points (in place of needles). More and more, research studies are documenting the ability of magnetic therapy to alleviate symptoms in a variety of conditions associated with chronic pain. Biomagnets have been used extensively by professional athletes with varying degrees of success, and increasingly by the general public who have heard about the good results by word of mouth. The medical community remains skeptical.

Magnetic therapy is used most often as a self-help procedure to ease a number of symptoms including chronic pain and sleep disturbances. Many fibromyalgia patients benefit from using biomagnets (a mattress pad, shoe inserts, and/or spot magnets) over specific problem areas. These are available from several sources. On average, I have seen a favorable response in 60 to 70 percent of patients who use biomagnets. This means that they notice a significant improvement in their symptoms—not that their symptoms are necessarily eliminated. Try to either borrow the biomagnets for a couple of weeks for a therapeutic trial or buy them from a reputable vendor who offers a 90-day money-back guarantee just in case you're in the 30- to 40-percent nonresponder group.

By the way, refrigerator door magnets will not work! Aside from differences in actual shape, size, and outward physical characteristics, biomagnets have been designed specifically with a strength (measured in Gauss) that falls within a biologic "therapeutic window." A typical strength range for biomagnets is from 400 to 4,000 Gauss. Weaker magnets aren't very effective; stronger magnets can be used but occasionally cause problems, such as impaired memory or concentration, when used near the head.

CAUTION—Don't use magnets if you're pregnant or if you have any implanted electrical device, such as a pacemaker, in your body (which could cause a potentially serious malfunction). In general, it's best to have a diagnosis and know what you're treating before using biomagnets. It is sometimes possible to mask the symptoms of a potentially life-threatening condition with the pain-relieving properties of biomagnets. If your symptoms worsen when using magnets, seek immediate medical attention.

ELECTROSTATIC MASSAGE

Electrostatic massage (EM) is a simple, noninvasive technique that uses static electricity to relieve certain types of pain. Respected research scientists have shown repeatedly that in the normal healing process, electrons flow to the abnormal area in what has been termed the "current of injury." Interfering with or enhancing the current of injury hinders or helps the healing process.

In electrostatic massage, a 12-inch section of ordinary Schedule 40 PVC pipe, 1 to 1 ½ inches in diameter, is given a negative electrical charge by rubbing it vigorously with a fuzzy or furry cloth (for example, a painter's mitt, available from any hardware store). The electrostatically-charged pipe is then moved over the treatment area, approximately ½ to 1 inch from the body, in a slow, sweeping motion, from top to bottom. Keep the pipe in motion until the symptoms have abated or 15 minutes have elapsed, whichever comes first. (Since the electrostatic charge diminishes with time, the pipe needs to be recharged with the painter's mitt after every three to six passes.)

This process pushes electrons to the symptomatic area and corrects charge imbalances associated with pathology. Because water is extremely responsive to electrostatic charge, EM can also reduce swelling or edema by drawing away the water that accumulates in an area of inflammation.

Although relief is short-term, I have used EM with considerable success on patients suffering from fibromyalgia, general muscular pain, arthritis, sinus and tension headaches, and tendinitis. Of 422 patients treated in my office with EM, 316 (75 percent) responded within five to 15 minutes, demonstrating either improved range of motion, decreased tenderness, or decreased pain. Twenty-five of these individuals had fibromyalgia, and 20 showed positive results.

Once you learn the technique, you can use it independently, thus reducing the need for expensive medical interventions. One drawback or limitation of this technique is that the vigorous rubbing motion required to generate the electrostatic charge may irritate your muscles, joints, and tendons. Some patients with osteoarthritis of the hands, carpal tunnel syndrome, or tendinitis of the hands/wrists/forearms may aggravate their underlying condition by this activity, or they might not have enough grip strength to generate adequate friction and charge (the PVC pipe will actually become hot from the friction). If you're unable to treat yourself, ask a friend to perform EM on you.

POLARITY THERAPY

Polarity therapy takes a holistic approach to treatment. A polarity therapist will work to balance your energy field by placing his or her hands on specific electrically charged points along your craniosacral system (the skull, spine, and sacrum or tail bone) to release their energy current. He or she can also teach you some self-help relaxation techniques you can use to balance your energy flow. The polarity practitioner may also recommend a course of treatment involving massage, breathing exercises, stretches, reflexology, or hydrotherapy.

Polarity yoga, based on the body's natural movements, is a series of postures designed to help maintain muscle tone, release toxins, and strengthen the spine. Two exercises that may offer some relief are the Relaxing Pose and the Calming Stretch.

Relaxing Pose

Sit for two minutes with the soles of your feet together. Gently push your knees upward and push against them with your hands. Keep the shoulders back to avoid slouching.

Calming Stretch

Sit on the floor with legs extended. Bend your knees slightly, keeping the heels of your feet on the floor. Bend from the hip and reach forward to grasp your toes. Hold for three minutes while gently rocking back and forth.

REIKI

Reiki is a Japanese form of energy healing developed in the mid-nineteenth century that seeks to heal your body, mind, and spirit. It is based on the philosophy that energy flows from the practitioner's hands into your energy field.

The Reiki practitioner places his or her hands over the energy centers (also known as *chakras*) of your body. Treatment often begins at the head, then moves to a specific part of the body where you are experiencing problems. The practitioner is thought to act as a conduit of energy from the environment by performing a sequence of hand movements that direct energy into your body's field.

Reiki practitioners believe the procedure causes the body's molecules to vibrate with higher intensity which in turn causes energy blockages to dissolve. When the blockages have been eliminated, harmony and health are facilitated. Changes are subtle at first and can include a sense of relief and relaxation, a release of anxiety and depression, and improved breathing. You may feel either invigorated or relaxed after a treatment.

The process of training to become a Reiki master used to take years. Now many practitioners become masters by taking a weekend seminar! Obviously, there can be huge differences in the skill levels of different practitioners, given the disparities in training and experience. Due to the lack of licensing standards in this discipline, it's important to rely on the practitioner's track record. Does he or she get results? (Ask the practitioner for the names of a few patients in an attempt to get a more unbiased appraisal.)

THERAPEUTIC TOUCH

Many fibromyalgia patients have found therapeutic touch helpful when it comes to coping with painful muscles. When muscles are tense, they build up lactic acid, which, in turn, makes them even more tense and painful.

In 1960 Dr. Dolores Krieger learned from healer Dora Kunz the technique of "laying on of hands" (which she had learned, in turn, from Charles Leadbeater and Oskar Estebany). During the 1970s Dr. Krieger taught what she called "therapeutic touch" to her graduate nursing students at New York University in an attempt to personalize the patient–nurse relationship. At least thirty thousand American nurses use this technique (or "healing touch" which is quite similar and derived from the same source) to attune their healing energy with the patient's in order to balance any disturbances in the patient's energy flow.

While there are research studies both supporting and refuting the clinical effects of therapeutic touch, many patients report benefits in the following areas:

- Relief of muscle spasms and tension.
- Relief of tension headaches and headaches associated with fibromyalgia.
- Strengthening of the immune system.
- Reduction of blood pressure.
- Improved digestion.
- Improved sense of calm.
- Relaxation of the nervous system and reduced anxiety.

9

Biochemical Approaches

HERBAL MEDICINE
AROMATHERAPY
NATUROPATHY

Your search for symptom relief may lead you to a number of complementary/alternative approaches that can be explained, at least in part, in terms of the effects they have on the body's biochemistry. This same biochemical model provides the foundation for Western or allopathic medicine. In its simplest form, the Western biomedical model sees the body in terms of anatomic structures and systems that are sustained by biochemical processes.

In this category, the major CAM therapies are nutritional and herbal. Nutritional approaches play such a major role in your general health and wellness that we've dealt with diet and supplementation in their own chapters. In this chapter, we'll take a close look at herbal medicine.

You'll also learn something about aromatherapy and naturopathic medicine. Naturopathic physicians also work, at least in part, within the biochemical model and take a multidisciplinary approach to diagnosis and treatment that can be very effective in managing fibromyalgia.

HERBAL MEDICINE

Herbs have been used in folk remedies around the world since ancient times. They were used in early Greek and Roman civilizations and were introduced to Europe during the Crusades. In the United States, herbs were used for many years to prevent illnesses and to treat minor complaints. Until the 1930s, in fact, herbs were the primary choice of many physicians in this country—for example, peppermint to soothe an upset stomach, garlic to prevent colds and flu.

As medical technology advanced and new pharmaceuticals were developed and marketed, the use of herbal remedies declined. Recently, however, there's been a renewed interest in natural botanicals, thanks in large part to the mounting expense of synthetic drugs and some of their serious side effects. Today, herbs are a booming business in the United States. In 1999, we spent an estimated $4.4 billion on natural plant remedies.

It's interesting to note that many common prescription and over-the-counter drugs were derived from herbs. Aspirin, for example, was originally developed from willow bark. Quinine, used to treat malaria, comes from the bark of an evergreen tree indigenous to South America and cultivated in hot climates. Taxol, a powerful drug used to combat breast cancer, comes from the Pacific yew tree. The painkiller morphine is derived from the opium poppy. Digitalis, a heart medication, is derived from foxglove.

It's usually safe to treat yourself with herbs for minor conditions. For colds, try some echinacea; for mild digestive complaints, sip a cup of peppermint tea. But even herbs that are generally safe need to be used with caution. By stimulating the immune system, echinacea can create problems for persons with autoimmune disease. Peppermint tea can bring discomfort to anyone suffering from heartburn or gastroesophageal reflux disease (GERD). High doses of licorice root can raise your blood pressure. Chamomile can trigger a reaction if you're allergic to ragweed. And too much ginger can cause gas, nausea, and vomiting—although in smaller doses it can ease those very same symptoms.

WHY SOME DOCTORS ARE SKEPTICAL ABOUT HERBS

Western-trained physicians are likely to be skeptical about claims made for herbal therapies. Many have ingrained doubts about the effectiveness of botanical remedies in general. Others admit they are simply not well enough informed to venture an opinion. A common complaint of physicians relates to multi-herb formulas. Doctors contend that when several herbs are combined in a single product targeted to a broad range of symptoms, it's impossible to evaluate in any scientific way which ingredients are acting on which symptom. Doctors also point out that many of the research studies cited by the manufacturers of herbal remedies are still not being published in peer-reviewed journals.

Critics of herbal therapy also contend, with some justification, that because herbal preparations are not regulated by the Food and Drug Administration (FDA) as pharmaceuticals are, potency can vary from brand to brand, even from bottle to bottle from the same manufacturer. With poor regulation of this industry and lack of universal standardization, herbs may be contaminated, adulterated, or otherwise of unknown quality. It's best to stick with well-known products from reputable companies.

SAFETY GUIDELINES FOR HERBAL THERAPY

If you're considering herbal therapy, first have your health problem diagnosed by a qualified practitioner. It's important to know exactly what you're treating so you can rule out a more serious condition which could require conventional drugs. Also, it's possible to mask the symptoms of a serious underlying condition with the use of natural remedies.

- It's always best to use herbs under the supervision of a health care practitioner who is familiar with herbal medicine. In the United States this might be a naturopath, a specialist in botanical medicine, an acupuncturist trained in Chinese herbalism, an Ayurvedic healer, or a trained medical or clinical herbalist.
- Herbal medicine is not a one-size-fits-all therapy. Your practitioner will devise a treatment strategy based on your condition and on your medical and family history. The type of preparation and the

dosage will depend on the strength of the herb, your age, and the results sought.

- Inform *all* of your health care practitioners about *all* the medicines and herbal preparations you're taking. Some herbs can cause allergic reactions or don't mix well with conventional drugs.

- Learn as much as you can about an herb before you take it. Are there side effects or warnings? How much and how often should you take it? Does it work best as a tablet or capsule, a tincture or tea?

- Avoid taking potentially toxic herbs, including chaparral, comfrey (taken orally), ephedra (ma huang), germander, Indian snakeroot, lobelia, pennyroyal, wormwood, and yohimbe.

- Buy from reputable manufacturers. In the past, European botanicals have tended to be of higher quality. Recently, however, several United States companies have introduced more stringent standards and now produce top-of-the-line botanical products.

- The FDA now requires herbal preparations to be labeled with the herb's scientific name, the amount of active ingredient(s), and the plant parts used. Product labels should also include the company's address, batch and lot numbers, expiration date, and dosage guidelines.

- Start with the lowest possible dose, and do not exceed the recommended dose. The toxicity of herbal products is largely untested.

- Don't pick herbs yourself from chemically treated lawns or gardens.
- In general, it's best to avoid herbs if you're pregnant.
- Consult a physician before taking herbs if you have allergies, are sensitive to drugs, or are taking prescription medications for chronic illness.
- Stop using herbal medicines two to three weeks before any scheduled surgery. Some herbs may have dangerous interactions with medications used during anesthesia or may increase the risk of bleeding complications.
- Consult a physician before giving herbs to children under 12 or to adults over 65.
- Be patient; herbs take longer to work than synthetic drugs. It may take six to eight weeks before you notice any benefits. However, the good news is that herbs retain their therapeutic strength over several years, so you won't need to keep increasing the dosage.
- If you experience any side effects, such as diarrhea or headache, stop taking the herb immediately and call your doctor. You can also call the FDA hotline at 800-332-1088.

MAKING HERBAL PREPARATIONS AT HOME

Having emphasized the need for standardized products, it would seem contradictory to suggest that you make your own herbal preparations. However, homemade preparations are perfectly safe for treating minor conditions. The

What to Look for on the Label

The phrase *caveat emptor* is particularly appropriate when it comes to purchasing nutritional and herbal supplements. In a recent study reported in the *New England Journal of Medicine* (1998), up to 25 percent of Chinese herbal supplements contained either significant contaminants (sometimes toxic levels of lead or arsenic), or unlabeled adulterants (such as cortisone) that were added to boost the effect of the labeled ingredients. Studies done by consumer groups, using independent laboratory assays, have found huge variations in the amount or percentage of active ingredients in nutritional products made by different manufacturers.

The virtual lack of regulation within the nutritional supplement industry forces wise consumers to seek out companies that voluntarily regulate themselves to control quality and meet high standards of safety. To judge whether a product is made by a responsible manufacturer, look for these important clues on the packaging:

Address and phone number—A mailing/e-mail address, Web site, or toll-free phone number should be provided for contacting the company with questions or problems.

Expiration date—Many supplements have a limited shelf life, and it's hard to know how long they've been sitting in a warehouse, in a store, or in a medicine cabinet before consumption. Discard supplements if past their expiration date.

FDA registration of manufacturing facilities—Some companies have had their facilities inspected and have submitted extensive documentation in order to secure FDA registration. This is good evidence that a manufacturer is not cutting corners.

GMP compliance—Voluntary adherence to Good Manufacturing Practices (GMP) is another sign that the company is behaving responsibly.

Independent laboratory assays—Anyone can make content claims on a label, but they should be able to prove these claims with objective, unbiased data. Independent laboratory verification of both the amount of active ingredients and the absence of contaminants or adulterants is important, but may not be documented on the packaging. Responsible manufacturers are able to readily provide this information on request.

Lot/Batch number—Product tracking through lot and batch numbers is vital for quality control purposes.

Milligrams of each ingredient per dose—Avoid products that have a long list of ingredients but give only the total milligram dosage. It should be clear how many milligrams or units of each ingredient are in each dose (capsule, tablet, dropper, or teaspoon).

Percentage of active ingredient—In many cases research has shown a certain percentage of a specific active ingredient is needed for clinical efficacy. If this type of research is available, then the manufacturer should meet that standard.

Recommended daily dose—You run the risk of both overdosing and underdosing without explicit instructions on the bottle.

Return policy—Reputable companies will refund your money if you're not satisfied with their product.

Side effects/Precautions—Responsible manufacturers warn consumers of contraindications to using their product, as well as potential interactions and side effects.

Product-specific research—Look for evidence of research done with that company's specific product and not something similar (you hope) made by a different manufacturer.

process can be fun and could save you some money. At worst, your homemade herbal preparations will be ineffective, requiring you to use a standardized product or even a prescription. In some cases, taking some time out of your hectic schedule to perform the healing ritual of making herbal preparations can be even more therapeutic than using the herb itself.

It's relatively easy to make a variety of herbal preparations including decoctions, tinctures, infusions, infused oils, creams, and ointments. Use infusions and decoctions within a day of preparation. Infused oils, creams, and ointments will last for several months, and tinctures last up to two years.

Make a *decoction* by boiling tough plant materials—such as bark, root, and berries—to extract their active ingredients. You can use fresh or dried herbs, alone or in combination. To prepare, place herbs in a saucepan, cover with cold water, and bring to a boil. Simmer until the liquid has been reduced by about one-third. Strain the liquid into a jar, then cover and store in a cool place. Drink decoctions hot or cold.

Prepare a *tincture* by soaking one or more herbs in alcohol and water for two weeks and then straining the mixture into a jar. Discard any herbs that are left after straining. Store in dark bottles for up to two years.

Infusions are similar to teas and can be drunk hot or cold. Place herbs—either alone or in combination—in a teapot and cover with boiling water. Cover the teapot and let the mixture steep for 10 minutes. Pour the infusion through a strainer into a cup, and add honey if you prefer a sweetened drink. Strain any remaining infusion into a jar. Cover and store in a cool place.

Infused oils are used for massage or in creams and ointments. Prepare hot infused oils by placing chopped herbs and oil in a glass bowl. Set the bowl in a pan of boiling water and simmer gently for two to three hours. Remove the mixture from the heat, cool, and strain. Pour the oil into dark glass bottles, seal, and store for up to a year. Use sunlight to prepare cold infused oils.

Skin creams are made by melting emulsifying wax in a glass bowl that has been set into a pan of boiling water. Add herbs, glycerin, and water, stir, and then simmer for about three hours. Strain the mixture using a piece of cheesecloth, then stir until it cools and sets. Place in a dark glass jar, seal with an airtight lid, and store in the refrigerator.

Ointments to protect the skin are made by placing olive oil and beeswax in a glass bowl set into a pan of boiling water. Add herbs and simmer for several hours. Strain the liquid through a piece of cheesecloth, into a dark glass jar. Seal the jar after the ointment has cooled and set.

Because so many people who use, sell, and recommend herbal therapies group them together with nutritional supplements (a bias encouraged by those in the nutritional supplement industry), you'll find specific information on herbal therapies that address the pain and fatigue of fibromyalgia in Chapter 5.

AROMATHERAPY

Aromatic oils, herbs, flowers, and other natural substances have been used since ancient Egyptian times for medicinal, cosmetic, and religious purposes. The modern scientific use of essential oils was discovered by French chemist Rene-Maurice Gattefosse, who worked in a perfume factory in the 1920s and coined the term aromatherapy.

The modality involves the therapeutic use of essential oils which are applied to the skin or inhaled. As these oils are absorbed into the body, most people experience a physiologic or biochemical effect. There is usually also a mind–body effect mediated through the olfactory nerve, triggering a strong emotional response via the limbic system—that part of our central nervous system that deals with strong emotions such as fear, joy, anger, and sexual desire. The limbic system, in turn, affects other parts of the brain which regulate such important functions as breathing, heart rate, and body temperature. There is even speculation that there may be an energetic effect related to the vibrational frequencies of the essential oils, although currently there is no research to support this concept.

The essential oils used in aromatherapy may be helpful for such conditions as menstrual irregularities, anxiety, arthritis, muscle aches, headaches, insomnia, psoriasis, insect stings, digestive problems, chest and nasal congestion, yeast infections, cystitis, and wound healing. There is currently no licensing process for aromatherapy practitioners in the United States.

The oils are sold in tiny, dark-tinted bottles in health food shops, holistic pharmacies, and through the mail. Buy from a reputable merchant and make sure the bottle is well-sealed and labeled "essential oil." Store in a cool place, away from the light.

Oils can be used by themselves or in combination, and can be inhaled from a cotton ball or handkerchief; misted into the air with a diffuser, humidifier, or vaporizer; diluted with a carrier oil and massaged into the skin; added to the bath; or added to a sachet to scent a drawer or closet.

Essential oils are intensely concentrated and highly potent. For inhalations, sprinkle four or five drops on a handkerchief, tissue, or cotton ball, hold to your nose, and take several deep breaths. You can also add a few drops to a bowl of steaming water, cover your head with a towel, lean over the bowl with your eyes closed, and inhale for up to 10 minutes. Do not inhale oils directly from the bottle.

To use oils in a vaporizer, place two or three drops in a bowl with a small amount of water and place over a lighted candle. You can also mist the room with a diffuser (sold where you buy your oils) or with a humidifier to which you've added several drops of oil.

For an aromatherapy bath, add six to eight drops of essential oil to a warm bath, and soak for at least 10 minutes.

CAUTION—Never use essential oils as a substitute for necessary medical care. Never use essential oils internally, near the eyes, or inhaled directly from the bottle. Essential oils should not be applied directly to the skin or mucous membranes full-strength, but should be diluted in a carrier oil such as apricot kernel oil, sunflower oil, or sweet almond oil. The customary formula is 10 drops of essential oil per 20 milliliter (ml) of carrier oil. For sensitive skin or if you are pregnant, use 5 drops per 20 ml. Make sure you're not allergic to the oil before using. Test yourself by applying a drop of diluted oil inside your elbow and waiting 24 hours. If a rash develops, discontinue use. Keep all essential oils out of the reach of children. If you have asthma, check with your physician before using essential oils.

RELIEF HAS NEVER SMELLED SO NICE!

To ease stiff, achy joints and muscles, try a warm (not hot) scented bath. Add 6 to 8 drops of essential oils of juniper, lavender, or rosemary (or 2 drops of each) to the water while the tub is filling, then relax in the warm bath for at least 15 minutes. If you're not in the mood for a soak, you can blend 4 to10 drops of essential oil per ounce of carrier oil and gently massage the diluted solution into the sore areas.

Clary sage and rose oils can lift your mood. Use these in a bath or inhale them from a handkerchief or cotton ball. You can also mist them into the air from a humidifier, vaporizer, or diffuser.

Lavender and peppermint oils, used alone or together, work well on headaches. Inhale, use a cool compress, or blend a few drops of the lavender oil with a carrier oil and rub a few drops on your temples, forehead, or back of the neck.

To help you sleep better, add neroli, lavender, and chamomile oil to the bath; all have sedative qualities and can promote sleep. Marjoram, sandalwood, juniper, and ylang ylang are also good for relaxation.

NATUROPATHY

Broadly trained in many modalities, naturopathic physicians (N.D.s) take an eclectic approach to natural healing, selecting those modalities that best stimulate the body's own innate healing responses. Naturopathic therapies may include nutritional interventions, mind–body techniques, homeothy, musculoskeletal manipulations, lifestyle modification, environmental medicine acupuncture, or herbal medicine.

Naturopathic practitioners stress holistic care and frequently treat conditions that are affected most by lifestyle and environment. Like Hippocrates, the father of modern medicine, they strive to do no harm by choosing treatments that are noninvasive and have few side effects. Every illness, they say, has an underlying cause. Treat the cause and the illness won't come back. For individuals with high blood pressure, treatment may involve a combination of diet, vitamins and minerals, herbs, and lifestyle changes. For arthritis sufferers, a regimen could involve diet, homeopathic medicines, acupuncture, hydrotherapy, and massage.

A visit to a naturopath will include a standard physical exam. The practitioner will take a medical history and ask questions about your lifestyle—including diet, exercise, stress, and emotional issues. Then the patient and practitioner work together to establish a treatment program that emphasizes lifestyle changes that can lead to better health. Naturopathy believes prevention is the best health strategy, and by changing unhealthy habits, you can avoid more serious problems in the future. For a specific complaint, the practitioner may prescribe one or more complementary therapies.

Licensing requirements for naturopathic doctors vary from state to state. While some states do not license naturopaths nor recognize their right to practice, in other states naturopaths are licensed to prescribe conventional medications, give vaccinations, and perform minor outpatient surgery. Most who have licenses have graduated from one of the three accredited schools of naturopathy in the United States: the National College of Naturopathic Medicine, Bastyr University, or the Southwest College of Naturopathic Medicine and Health Sciences.

Graduates of these schools belong to the American Association of Naturopathic Physicians (AANP). Naturopaths follow a pre-med course as undergraduates, followed by four years of graduate school. They study such traditional medical subjects as anatomy, histology, pharmacology, and pathology, as well as naturopathic philosophy, Chinese medicine, nutrition, hydrotherapy, and other complementary therapies. They also work in a clinical setting with a licensed naturopath before obtaining an N.D. degree.

The American Naturopathic Medical Association (ANMA) is a competing organization, and its members typically have not attended a four-year naturopathic college. Many, but not all, ANMA members have prior biomedical training as nurses, pharmacists, or physicians, and they've taken a shorter training program (sometimes by correspondence).

The two organizations have been waging a political battle for many years over who is a "true naturopath" (and who, therefore, qualifies for licensure and insurance recognition). AANP members typically paint ANMA members as inferior, unqualified practitioners who bought their diplomas from correspondence diploma mills. ANMA members often portray AANP members as power-grabbing, M.D. wannabes who have betrayed the naturopathic profession.

In my experience neither characterization is fair since I've found both exceptional and marginal practitioners in each camp. When the two organizations quit fighting long enough to agree to a national certification exam that applies equally to everyone (no matter where the person was trained), it will be far easier for the general public to distinguish between credible and questionable naturopaths. A well-trained naturopathic physician is a pleasure to work with and is a font of knowledge regarding natural health and healing.

10
Structural Therapies

CHIROPRACTIC
OSTEOPATHY
CRANIOSACRAL THERAPY
TRIGGER POINT THERAPY
MASSAGE
BOWEN THERAPY
REFLEXOLOGY
HYDROTHERAPY

If you have fibromyalgia, sooner or later you will make your way to one or more of the complementary/alternative practitioners who specialize in musculoskeletal treatments, the so-called structural therapies. The effect of these interventions can be understood chiefly in terms of what they do to the anatomic structures of the body—the bones, muscles, ligaments, organs, and joints.

CAM practitioners working in this category include chiropractors, osteopaths, naturopaths, massage therapists, and hydrotherapists. These last two, along with physical therapists, fit very comfortably in the conventional medical framework as well, although individual practitioners often take a more holistic approach to treatment.

Reflexologists are often grouped in this category because, to untrained Western eyes, reflexology seems to be nothing more than foot or hand massage. Practitioners of the art would disagree, maintaining that the goal of treatment is to increase energy flow and restore energy balance.

CHIROPRACTIC

Chiropractic is a century-old healing art form that emphasizes the prevention of chronic disease through the maintenance of a healthy neuromusculoskeletal system. The specialty dates back to 1895 when Dr. Daniel David Palmer apparently was able to cure a patient's deafness by pushing a vertebra in the man's back into proper alignment. Palmer took this as proof that spinal misalignment could lead to health problems and that spinal realignment could restore the flow of nerve impulses throughout the body.

Chiropractors may use medical diagnostic procedures, including, but not limited to, x-rays of the spine, to assess dysfunction. They then use a combination of spinal manipulation and exercise to adjust the spinal column, correct structural imbalances, and restore range of motion. Some chiropractors also incorporate nutritional therapy, acupuncture, and other techniques into their practice.

Chiropractic care can offer pain relief without the use of drugs or surgery. Many patients find it an effective way to manage lower back pain, tension and migraine headaches, and neck problems. It also can complement traditional medical treatment for such long-term disorders as asthma, ringing in the ears, dizziness, and chronic fatigue syndrome.

During an office visit, a chiropractor will take your medical history, ask you about your lifestyle and symptoms, and evaluate your posture and walk. During the examination, he will feel your vertebrae and joints and may perform a reflex test to check for nerve function. He will ask you to bend forward, backward, and sideways to check your range of motion. He may order x-rays to determine if there are any underlying joint problems that could be made worse by treatment.

Once a diagnosis is made, the chiropractor will adjust your joints by means of a controlled push that moves the joint beyond its restricted range of motion. Treatments are painless, and many people see results in nine to 12 sessions.

Today there are more than fifty thousand chiropractors in the United States. More than twenty million people a year visit a chiropractor, making this the most popular form of nontraditional therapy (after the use of herbal and nutritional supplements).

Many physicians, however, continue to be skeptical of chiropractic care for any condition other than back pain and minor muscle and joint pain. These doubters maintain that chiropractors don't have the training to diagnose or treat any other conditions and could misdiagnose or prevent a patient from getting necessary medical treatment as quickly as possible. A competent chiropractor will, however, refer a patient to a medical doctor if symptoms warrant.

As college undergraduates, chiropractors follow a pre-med course of study for at least two years, followed by four years at an accredited chiropractic college. The curriculum is similar to the medical school curriculum, with additional emphasis on anatomy, nutrition, physiology, and rehabilitation. Chiropractors are licensed to practice in all 50 states and in the District of Columbia. To be licensed, they must be graduates of an accredited chiropractic college and must pass a rigorous exam. Chiropractors maintain their licenses by taking continuing education courses.

CAUTION—Chiropractic manipulation can cause severe damage in cases involving an underlying, unidentified fracture or tumor. If you have atherosclerosis of the carotid arteries, you should avoid vigorous manipulation of the neck as there is a small but distinct chance of dislodging some plaque and causing a stroke.

OSTEOPATHY

Osteopathy, or osteopathic medicine, dates back to the 1870s, to frontier doctor Andrew Taylor Still who believed that a person's bones, muscles, ligaments, and connective tissues—the musculoskeletal system—was the basis for good health. Based on this belief, Dr. Still created a system of healing that employed touch and gentle manipulation of muscles and joints to trigger the body's own ability to heal itself, often without drugs or surgery.

Osteopathic physicians gear their treatment toward three objectives: relieving tension so that muscles, ligaments, and joints are properly aligned; improving blood circulation and stimulating the nervous system; and correcting posture and other body mechanics to prevent health problems.

In addition to performing a complete physical exam with standard lab tests, an osteopath will conduct a structural exam to evaluate your posture, spine, and balance. She'll press on your muscles, tendons, and ligaments to see if you feel tenderness, tension, or weakness, and she'll evaluate your joints to assess your range of motion.

If a structural problem is found, the osteopath will use osteopathic manipulative therapy (OMT) that can involve massage, stretching, muscle pressure, and joint alignment. OMT is designed to relieve tension in affected muscles and ligaments, improve posture and movement, and promote better circulation to stimulate the body's own natural healing ability. It has been shown to work well for people with chronic pain (including lower back pain, headaches, and migraines), menstrual pain, and knee and neck problems.

While chiropractors usually limit their treatment to the spine, osteopaths may also work on the arms, legs, and skull in an effort to improve blood circulation, which is essential to healing. Some osteopaths may also recommend a regimen of treatment that can include acupuncture, massage therapy, or homeopathy, based on your individual symptoms. For acute illnesses and for those not caused by a structural abnormality, osteopaths often rely on conventional medical techniques, including drugs and surgery.

Doctors of osteopathy (D.O.s) are licensed as physicians in all 50 states and can prescribe medication. They undergo the same training as M.D.s in terms of basic and clinical sciences. They must be graduates of a four-year accredited college of osteopathy and must complete a one-year internship in primary care. Many osteopaths also complete a residency in one of 120 medical specialties. Medical boards make no distinction between D.O.s and M.D.s when it comes to standards of medical practice. The main difference is that osteopathic doctors have additional training in musculoskeletal diagnosis and manipulation. Not all D.O.s incorporate OMT into their practice, but those who do often have a more holistic approach to treating patients.

CRANIOSACRAL THERAPY

Developed by osteopath John Upledger at Michigan State University in the late 1970s, craniosacral therapy (sometimes called craniosacral release, or CSR) is a gentle, noninvasive method of evaluating and enhancing the function of the craniosacral system. It is thought that imbalances in this system—consisting of the membranes and fluids that run along the spinal cord from the cranium (skull) to the sacrum (tailbone)—can impede the normal flow of cerebrospinal fluid which carries nutrients throughout the central nervous system. Osteopaths, chiropractors, and massage therapists who use this technique lightly palpate these structures, detect the imbalances, and subtly adjust the bones. In doing so, they attempt to remove energy blockages and re-establish healthy flow, thus relieving the negative effects of stress and encouraging the body's natural healing mechanisms. In fibromyalgia patients, the flow is thought to be out of sync.

Craniosacral therapy has been used successfully to treat a variety of conditions including chronic pain, recurrent ear infections, head and neck injuries, eye difficulties, motor coordination impairments, headaches, hyperactivity, and emotional trauma.

TRIGGER POINT THERAPY

Trigger point therapy (also known as triggerpoint myotherapy) was developed by physical fitness expert Bonnie Prudden. It focuses on the trigger points, those tender, congested spots on muscles, tendons, and fascia that radiate pain to other areas of the body. The therapist locates the trigger points by pressing along a muscle and then applies pressure to these locations in order to relieve tension, relax muscle spasms, improve circulation, and decrease pain. The process itself can be uncomfortable, so it's important to communicate to the therapist in order to keep the pain to a minimum.

Using their knuckles, fingers, or elbows, trigger point therapists apply pressure directly to a trigger point for several seconds. The pressure breaks the pain-signal pattern that communicates between the brain and the muscle. Once that pattern is interrupted, the muscle relaxes. The therapist will then use a series of exercises to keep the muscle pain-free by developing healthy function. Clients are taught to avoid pain-producing postures and to stretch and strengthen their muscles.

Trigger point therapists are certified after undergoing a nine-month, 1,400-hour training program, a board examination, and 45 hours of continuing education credits every other year.

MASSAGE

You know how good a massage feels. But do you know the health benefits it delivers? Massage, the manipulation of soft tissues, may not cure what ails you, but it can go a long way toward relieving certain symptoms, particularly those caused by stress. A good massage helps you relax. It can also be effective in the treatment of sports-related injuries, muscle and joint problems, headaches, and chronic pain—even sinus problems and digestive difficulties. A therapeutic massage changes your physiology in ways that facilitate the normal healing process.

Massage can stretch tissues, increase your range of motion, help lower blood pressure and heart rate, and improve breathing. It can also be helpful in improving circulation, relaxing muscles, and eliminating the buildup of lactic acid in the muscles. Researchers believe massage helps the brain produce endorphins, the chemicals that act as natural painkillers.

A study published in the *Scandinavian Journal of Rheumatology* reported that 21 of 26 fibromyalgia patients experienced reduced pain and general improvement after receiving massage therapy. According to researchers, there is a relationship between the degree of pain a fibromyalgia patient feels and an increase in blood levels of myoglobin (the oxygen-carrying protein of the muscle tissue). The pain may result from the leakage of myoglobin from the muscles. The study showed that in addition to experiencing less pain after massage, the patients had a lower level of myoglobin in their blood.

Massage can certainly be helpful when it comes to easing pain, improving circulation, relaxing muscles, and eliminating the buildup of lactic acid in the muscles. For individuals with fibromyalgia, however, massage therapy has to start off gently, as strenuous massage can trigger flare-ups of muscular pain and actually make the condition worse. Generally, you want your massage therapist to stay on the lighter and more superficial side. The therapist will try to mobilize fluid and break up knotty trigger points in the tissues. These are stagnant areas; the wastes are not leaving, and the nutrients are not coming in. But you don't want the massage to be so aggressive that it triggers even more spasms, because these are very sensitive areas. As muscles become more relaxed, deeper massage can sometimes be used.

A specific type of massage, known as *myofascial release*, may be particularly helpful in treating chronic pain or in restoring range of motion. In this technique, the therapist uses a gentle, sustained pressure to soften up the connective tissue—known as the fascia—that surrounds bones, muscles, nerves, and internal organs and tissues. The fascia runs from head to toe in one continuous sheet; for that reason, the pain you feel in one part of your body may be caused by tension in a spot far removed from the site of your discomfort.

Your first few massage sessions may leave you exhausted as the toxins and blockages in your body are released into your bloodstream. Since your kidneys and liver will be working overtime to rid your body of these waste products, help them along by drinking lots of pure water, avoiding alcohol and cigarette smoke—even secondhand smoke—and eating light, nutritious meals.

Your body may be sore the day after a massage, but the discomfort should disappear quickly, usually by the following day. If not, tell the therapist to be more gentle next time.

CAUTION—While massage is generally safe for most people, consult your health care practitioner if you have heart disease, circulatory problems, cancer, an infectious illness, or a skin condition. Massage enhances lymphatic and blood flow, and even though there is no research documenting problems, there is a theoretic concern that it may thus facilitate bleeding and the spread of infection or localized tumor cells. If there is a localized problem area, it's best to avoid massage in that part of the body.

BOWEN THERAPY

Bowen therapy practitioners work on trigger point locations and acupressure points using a light touch with a rolling motion of their fingers and thumbs on any misaligned muscle. The touch signals the nerves beneath to cue the brain to move the muscle to its natural location. Treatments are believed to improve circulation, increase mobility, and promote the release of waste products from the tissues.

Treatments may last once a week for a month and then be scheduled monthly for six months. Muscles may take five to 10 days to respond after being treated. To find a qualified Bowen therapist, call the Blue River Institute at 413-665-3492.

Also Worth Investigating

There are many other structural interventions and techniques which we can't do justice to in the limited space of this book. Examples of some of these including Rolfing (also known as structural integration), soft tissue release (STR), neuromuscular technique (NMT), and *tui na* (Chinese medical massage).

REFLEXOLOGY

Reflexology, sometimes referred to as "zone therapy," has been practiced in one way or another for centuries. Reflexology is based on the idea that reflex points on the feet, hands, and ears correspond to activity elsewhere in the body. Manipulating specific reflex points stimulates the natural healing response in the corresponding parts of the body.

Your toes, for example, correspond to your head and neck. Your heel corresponds to your pelvic area, and so on. Pressure on corresponding points may cause soreness or tenderness. The more tenderness you feel, say reflexologists, the greater the need to balance your energy in that area. While most Westerners characterize this modality as a form of massage, reflexologists feel it is an energy-based intervention that promotes overall health by helping to correct energy imbalances.

Practitioners say the treatment improves blood circulation, balances overactive or underactive glands, and relieves stress. Daily treatment is thought to balance the body's energy, enhance relaxation, and help you stay healthy. The technique is also used to treat a number of ailments including insomnia, headaches, premenstrual syndrome, sinusitis, and constipation.

A skilled reflexologist can help you tackle sleep problems by concentrating on the points on your hands and feet related to the adrenal glands, diaphragm, parathyroid, pituitary, reproductive system, and spine. A reflexology session performed by a qualified practitioner can be one of the most relaxing experiences you've ever had.

Reflexology can be performed by a professional practitioner or you can try it yourself or with a partner. Learn which points to work on by visiting a trained reflexologist or by consulting self-help books.

Reflexologists are not licensed, but many are certified by the International Institute of Reflexology.

The basic technique is called "thumb walking" and involves using the inside edge of the thumb pad or the index finger in a slow, forward movement, bending the first joint of the thumb or finger slightly as it moves ahead. Hold your foot with one hand—the sole flat and the toes straight—and work on it with the other hand. To work on the hands, use the thumb of one hand on the palm of the other, or the index finger on the areas between the fingers. Feel for tension or gritty spots beneath the skin, known as "crystals." These are believed to be signs of the blockage causing your individual symptoms.

- For headaches, work on the points that correspond to your head, eyes, and ears. These points are found on your fingers and fingertips.
- For stress, concentrate on your hands by applying pressure up and down the outer edge of your thumb, from below the nail to your wrist.
- For shoulder and neck pain, massage the area that corresponds to the neck, which is located where the big toe joins the foot on the sole of the left foot. You can also massage the cervical spine area, located along the inner side of both feet, along the joint of the big toe. Or try rotating the big toe.

HYDROTHERAPY

Hydrotherapy—the use of water to relieve symptoms of health problems—can be traced to many ancient cultures, among them the Romans, Egyptians, and Hebrews. Native Americans used sweat lodges for cleansing and for ceremonial purposes. For many centuries, Scandinavians have used saunas to detoxify the blood after long winters without fresh food.

Water has been used internally and externally in a variety of treatment applications, including whirlpool baths, ice packs, saunas, douches, colonic irrigation, sitz baths, compresses, wraps, and mineral drinking waters.

Hot water treatments can relax muscles and increase joint mobility. Cold water treatments can be effective for pain relief and for reducing inflammation. Alternating hot and cold treatments (called "contrast therapy") can increase blood circulation through the elimination organs (the kidneys, liver, and skin), thereby detoxifying the system and improving the quality of the blood.

For some people with fibromyalgia, hot water can ease pain by soothing aching joints and relaxing sore muscles. For others, particularly those with myofascial muscle pain, heat can bring more fluids to the painful area and aggravate the condition. You have to experiment a bit and see what works best for you. If a hot soak in a tub or whirlpool, or a hot shower brings relief, keep the water no hotter than 110 degrees Fahrenheit (40 degrees Celsius) and don't stay in for more than 15 minutes. If hot baths seem to help, hot packs and heating pads may also provide relief.

Cold (ice) therapy can also be helpful in easing pain, especially for those with trigger point referred pain. Wrap the ice in a plastic bag and apply to the affected area in a 20-minutes-on, 20-minutes-off pattern. Applications should not exceed 20 minutes, as extended exposure to extreme cold can damage the skin.

Contrast therapies, which alternate between hot and cold water, may ease pain and increase circulation to an affected area. The heat relaxes, the cold stimulates. The contrast between the two improves your circulation, carrying more nutrients to your cells and ridding them more quickly of waste material. Applying heat to one part of the body while applying cold to another, moves blood from the cold area to the hot, and often helps ease pain in the cold region.

When alternating between hot and cold, don't use hot water for more than five or 10 minutes at a time; keep the cold water to just a few minutes. Always end with the cold.

11
Movement Therapies

YOGA
TAI CHI
QIGONG
ALEXANDER TECHNIQUE
FELDENKRAIS METHOD
TRAGER APPROACH

A program of regular, gentle exercise—one tailored to your capacities and limitations—can help you feel your best, even on days when your muscles are weak and painful. In this chapter, you'll find information on a number of exercise activities drawn from the complementary and alternative side of the menu.

The advantage of the CAM approaches is that they are particularly gentle on the body and are designed to address the whole person—body and mind—in a relaxing, restorative program of physical and mental fitness.

YOGA

Yoga, a Sanskrit word meaning "union," originated in India more than five thousand years ago. The practice of yoga is designed to quiet the mind by teaching you how to pay attention to your breathing and to the movement—or stillness—of your body.

The most popular form of yoga in Western culture is hatha-yoga, which focuses on the mind–body balance and uses physical postures known as *asanas*, breathing techniques, and meditation. By helping establish the proper alignment of energy within the body, yoga promotes general good health in the individuals who practice it.

The practice of yoga is undergoing a huge burst of popularity among baby boomers who are seeking gentler forms of exercise after years of bone-jarring aerobics and jogging.

Yoga experts recommend that you perform the yoga postures at least 30 minutes each day, preferably in the morning or late evening, on an empty stomach. Wear loose clothing. Start with several minutes of deep breathing to calm your mind and increase the flow of oxygen within your body. Follow with several warm-up exercises, and then move on to the postures you have chosen for that day. Perform each pose slowly and gently; the *asanas* should not cause pain.

End each session with the corpse pose and hold for five to 10 minutes of relaxation. For this pose, lie on your back with your feet about 18 inches apart and turned out slightly. Place your hands about 6 inches from your hips, palms up. Close your eyes and breathe deeply.

Yoga postures re-establish structural integrity by stretching and strengthening muscles to expand the natural range of motion, massage internal organs, relax nerves, and increase blood circulation. Depending on which poses you use, yoga can work on every muscle, nerve, and gland in your body. And because it focuses and calms the mind, it can help ease feelings of anxiety, fatigue, and depression, preventing or alleviating many stress-related conditions.

Yoga is useful not only as a stress-reducer but as a way to ease back and neck problems and relieve symptoms associated with heart disease, high blood pressure, arthritis, asthma, chronic fatigue syndrome, allergies, diabetes, and digestive problems. Integrated with a swimming and walking program, yoga can provide all the targeted exercise you need for flexibility, heart health, and strong bones.

Many people with fibromyalgia find the gentle movements and relaxing breathing exercises of yoga beneficial when it comes to managing pain and stiffness as well as relieving fatigue. Tense muscles hurt, and in turn cause painful joints to hurt even worse. Yoga postures can help stretch and strengthen the muscles in your back, shoulders, abdomen, hips, and legs. The breathing exercises and meditation that accompany yoga movements promote relaxation, which reduces pain even more. Yoga is also invigorating; if you do yoga exercises in the morning, you will have more energy to get through your day.

Although yoga is often practiced by followers of the Hindu religion, yoga itself is not a religion and can be

Two Yoga Poses to Try

These two *asanas* are just a sample of some of the poses that can be incorporated into a yoga routine:

Mountain Pose

The Mountain Pose teaches correct posture and is the basis for all other standing poses. Stand with your feet together so your big toes are touching and your heels are slightly apart. Let your arms hang freely at your sides. Spread and lengthen your toes. Lift your kneecaps so they are facing forward. Keep your pelvis balanced on your legs. Lengthen your spine by stretching your inner legs upward from the inner heels to the groin. Continue to lengthen upward, opening your chest. Drop your shoulders and lengthen the back of your neck. Relax your face, your throat, and your eyes. Hold this pose for up to one minute.

Standing Forward Bend

The standing forward bend restores your energy and invigorates you. Stand in the Mountain Pose one foot away from a wall with your knees slightly bent, your feet hip-width apart, and your back to the wall. Place your hands on the wall and rest your buttocks against it. Now place your hands on your hips and inhale. Exhale slowly, and bend forward from the hips. Bend your arms and clasp your elbows. Let your upper body hang down as you relax your neck and head, as well as your throat and eyes. Hold the pose for 20 seconds; gradually increase the time to one minute. Release your arms slowly, inhale, and return to the Mountain Pose.

practiced by people of all religions and philosophies. It was developed by spiritual students who wanted to strengthen and energize their bodies to better withstand the rigors of lengthy meditation. Classes are taught at health clubs, colleges, hospitals, and community centers. There are also a number of self-help books and videos that can teach you the basics.

Yoga instructors are not licensed. Some organizations do offer certification, but the requirements differ from group to group.

TAI CHI

For thousands of years, people in China have practiced *tai chi*, which combines physical and mental exercises in an effort to restore energy and vitality to both your body and mind. The exercises consist of a series of slow, flowing, rhythmic movements accompanied by deep breathing and can be performed by virtually anyone, regardless of age or physical condition. Millions of Chinese and Taiwanese people begin their day with a *tai chi* session performed en masse in local parks.

When performing *tai chi*, you move your arms through a series of slow, controlled, and continuous circles while shifting your weight from one foot to the other. The movements and positions are known as "forms" and have such names as Salutation to the Buddha, Grasp Bird's Tail, White Crane Spreads Its Wings, and Embracing Tiger.

Tai chi has been shown to reduce stress—as well as improve breathing, posture, and balance—by emphasizing complete relaxation. A 1998 study at the Johns Hopkins School of Medicine reported that *tai chi* exercises lowered blood pressure in older adults just as well as moderate aerobic exercise did.

Tai chi is recommended by the Arthritis Foundation for arthritis sufferers, because it emphasizes total relaxation and passive concentration with no risk of injury. Those who find exercise painful may find that *tai chi* enables them to slowly move their body through a full range of motion.

Although you can perform *tai chi* alone once you've mastered the exercises, you will need to find a good teacher to get started. To locate an instructor in your area, contact the American Oriental Bodywork Therapy Association at 856-782-1616 or look in the telephone book under "*tai chi*," "martial arts," "self-defense," "health services," and "holistic centers and/or practitioners."

QIGONG

Qigong exercises involve gentle, rhythmic swinging postures, stretching movements, meditation, and deep-relaxation breathing, with the objective of increasing the body's vital energy and calming the emotions and the mind. The slow-paced exercises stretch ligaments and tendons and flex muscles. A technique that involves remaining still for an extended period—from several minutes to an hour—is designed to teach concentration and enhance sensitivity to the flow of your energy. The regular practice of *qigong* can result in improved circulation, balance, flexibility, and increased range of motion. The exercises also improve overall relaxation.

To find a qualified *qigong* instructor, contact the American Oriental Bodywork Therapy Association at 856-782-1616, or look in the telephone book under "*qigong*," "*chigong*," "*chi kung*," or "*qi gung*." Holistic/wellness centers may also offer classes.

ALEXANDER TECHNIQUE

Individuals with fibromyalgia frequently experience shoulder and neck pain, which is often exacerbated by unconsciously adjusting their posture in an effort to cope with their discomfort. During Alexander "lessons," the student lies on a massage table while the teacher gently adjusts the student's body position, for instance, by moving the shoulders into their natural position. The Alexander technique teaches you how to reduce tension and strain on your muscles and joints. Practitioners believe it improves range of motion and enhances posture, balance, and coordination. Alexander teachers show you how to move without strain, based on the philosophy of founder F. M. Alexander: "Free the neck; let the neck go forward and upward; let the back lengthen and widen." The teacher will help you rethink your body movements and teach you how to avoid motions that can lead to muscle tension.

The Alexander teacher will first observe you lying on a table, fully clothed. He or she will then watch as you stand, walk, and perform routine tasks. Lessons are usually given on a one-on-one basis, and run from 30 minutes to an hour, once a week for a minimum of 15 weeks.

FELDENKRAIS METHOD

Feldenkrais was developed by Dr. Moshe Feldenkrais, a nuclear physicist, an avid soccer player, and a judo expert who earned the first black belt in judo awarded in the Western hemisphere. He also developed a system of somatic education that raises student awareness of unconscious, ingrained movement habits.

The system is taught in two parts. *Awareness Through Movement* involves group lessons in light, effortless movements that focus primarily on how you move. *Functional Integration* involves one-on-one lessons that usually include gentle, directive touch to suggest a greater repertoire of movement possibilities that translate to your central nervous system.

Feldenkrais created thousands of ingenious lessons aimed at improving the quality of movement, thought, and behavior for people with certain chronic and acute injuries, stroke, and restrictions due to age. People report improvement in posture, breathing, coordination, and sensitivity with the use of this gentle, noninvasive method. Many have reported reduction or elimination of chronic neuromuscular pain, an enhancement of mental and physical abilities, and improved general well-being.

Feldenkrais can also be used to help individuals with disorders such as cerebral palsy and multiple sclerosis.

TRAGER APPROACH

The Trager approach is a form of movement re-education that is made up of a series of gentle, passive movements and rotation and traction of the limbs. Movements are adjusted to each individual's condition so that tightness and stiffness can be released without pain. This system was developed by physician Milton Trager in the 1920s to help polio victims and others suffering from neuro-muscular conditions.

The Trager practitioner will move your limbs through smooth joint movements. He or she will then gently and rhythmically rock each part of the body in order to show you how free and easy movement can be. As you experience these feelings, the nerves that control muscle movement will register this information to reorganize and release patterns of tension, pain, and muscle restriction. The rocking also promotes deep relaxation. No force or pressure is used. The practitioner will also teach simple movements—called mentastics—for you to do at home. These movements will help recreate the feelings experienced during the session and are designed to increase energy levels and improve mobility. Participants say that with practice, the Trager approach can help relieve chronic pain and promote joint mobility, deeper states of relaxation, heightened levels of energy and vitality, and more effortless posture.

Trager practitioners are certified after completing a six-month program at the Trager Institute in Mill Valley, California.

12
Mind–Body Therapies

BIOFEEDBACK
DEEP ABDOMINAL BREATHING
MEDITATION
GUIDED IMAGERY
HYPNOTHERAPY
PRAYER
LOVE AND LAUGHTER
PET THERAPY

Mind–body medicine is a broad field encompassing many different mental techniques or therapies that have been shown to alter physiology. For the fibromyalgia patient, a number of these techniques or therapies are relevant treatment strategies. Examples of some mind–body therapies include biofeedback, EMDR (eye movement desensitization reprogramming), guided imagery, meditation, hypnotherapy, laughter therapy, music therapy, pet therapy, and behavioral therapy (counseling).

Stress reduction is a primary goal of these interventions. The typical physical responses associated with the mind–body therapies include reduced blood pressure, reduced blood clotting, elevated endorphins (which relieve pain and give a feeling of well-being), reduced levels of cortisol and adrenaline (stress hormones that lower immunity and alter circulation), reduced muscle tension, and improved circulation.

Some of the conditions that have responded favorably to mind–body interventions include allergies, angina, anxiety, asthma, back pain, depression, headaches, hypertension, irritable bowel syndrome, post-traumatic stress disorder (PTSD), and Raynaud's disease. As you know, some of these disorders are also present in cases of fibromyalgia.

Stress is a significant issue for anyone with fibromyalgia, because anxiety and tension can trigger a flare-up of symptoms. Of course, no one lives a stress-free existence, but we can all learn to do a better job of managing stress. In addition to the lifestyle changes suggested in Chapter 6, you may want to explore one or more of the mind–body approaches. We are just starting to grasp how powerful these therapies are for anyone dealing with the near-constant stress of long-term illness.

BIOFEEDBACK

Biofeedback uses a variety of devices to measure physical changes that signal the body's state of stress or relaxation. Normally, these internal processes—including heart rate, skin temperature, galvanic skin response (a measure of electrical conductivity), blood pressure, and even brain waves—go unnoticed, but when we are made aware of them through the aid of specialized equipment, we can learn various techniques to consciously control them.

Such techniques include the use of imagery, breathing, and progressive muscle relaxation. After some practice with biofeedback, you can become aware of your various body processes without the aid of equipment. Then you can use the relaxation techniques you've learned to dial down anxiety and keep your body in a more relaxed state while dealing with the demands and stresses of daily life.

Since the 1960s researchers have accumulated an impressive body of research confirming the therapeutic value of biofeedback. It has been used successfully to treat a number of stress-related conditions such as high blood pressure, anxiety, insomnia, tension headaches, migraines, irritable bowel syndrome, chronic back pain, and Raynaud's disease. As biofeedback becomes more mainstream, it's proving to be a very useful therapeutic tool.

Biofeedback has also been shown to be an effective mind–body approach for people with fibromyalgia. In fibromyalgia patients, blood circulation to the muscles of the back, arms, legs, hands, and feet is frequently compromised. Using biofeedback, you can literally retrain your blood vessels to dilate when necessary, to increase circulation to a specific body part.

Biofeedback can also be used to restore normal function to the diaphragm, which will improve breathing and reduce stress on the muscles of the neck and upper chest.

Through biofeedback, you can also learn which activities cause you to "overdo," and you can modify your behavior as a result. Once you learn your body's natural patterns, you can work to adjust them for better relaxation and sounder sleep.

In one study, 15 fibromyalgia patients who had not responded well to medication were trained with biofeedback. After 15 sessions, they reported fewer tender points, less pain, and some relief from morning stiffness.

The most common type of biofeedback used in medical settings is electromyographic (EMG) biofeedback, which measures electrical activity in muscles. The procedure is painless, and people quickly get the hang of it. Electrodes can be attached to several sites on your body to monitor blood pressure, skin temperature, and other biological functions and/or neuromuscular activity. The responses are then interpreted, and the practitioner teaches you how to alter your mental and emotional states for healthier, less stressful functioning. Once you learn the basic techniques, you can use them to modify your responses at any time and in any place.

DEEP ABDOMINAL BREATHING

Deep abdominal breathing is one of the stress-reduction techniques that can help you learn to relax, and in turn, ease anxiety and promote more restful sleep.

When you learn to control your breathing, you can decrease the release of stress hormones in your body and slow your heart rate. Often people who are under stress will hyperventilate, taking quick, shallow breaths that move the upper chest more than the abdomen. This type of breathing is not only inefficient, it is also counterproductive and leads to even more physical and mental stress. Deep abdominal breathing can cause your body to release endorphins, those natural body chemicals that promote a sense of well-being.

To practice deep breathing, lie on your back in a quiet room with no distractions. Place your hands on your abdomen and breathe in slowly and deeply through your nostrils. If you are breathing correctly, your hands will rise as your abdomen expands. Inhale to a count of five, hold your breath for three seconds, then exhale to a count of five. Note the coolness of the air as it enters your nostrils and the warmth of the air as you exhale. Do this exercise 10 times at first, increasing to 25 times, twice a day.

When you get the hang of deep breathing, you can combine it with progressive muscle relaxation. This technique involves contracting and relaxing all the muscle groups in the body, one at a time.

Find a quiet place where you won't be disturbed. Sit comfortably with your feet flat on the floor, your back straight, and your hands resting on your thighs. Do not cross your feet, legs, arms, or hands. Close your eyes, and as soon as you are comfortable, begin to focus on your breathing. Take a few deep breaths, allowing your chest and abdomen to expand with each breath.

Now begin to focus on relaxing each part of your body, beginning with your feet, moving upward to your calves, your thighs, then to your fingers, hands, wrists, forearms, and upper arms. Allow each part of your body to go limp and heavy, as if you were going to melt into the chair and floor. Next relax your stomach muscles, then your chest. Move on to your lower back, upper back, and shoulders. Finally relax the back of your neck, your face, your throat, and the muscles of your jaw. Once you're completely relaxed, you're ready to meditate.

MEDITATION

Meditation can help relax your body and mind. While the practice is used as a pathway to spiritual enlightenment in Eastern cultures, in the West meditation is used in a nonreligious context to promote peace of mind and ease stress-related symptoms such as chronic pain, high blood pressure, panic disorders, headaches, respiratory problems, insomnia, and premenstrual syndrome.

Practicing meditation every day can help you focus on your healing and ease the stress of living with fibromyalgia. Meditation can move you into a calmer, more relaxed state by slowing your heart rate and breathing, lowering your blood pressure, relaxing your muscles, and clearing your mind. Slow, deep breathing accompanies each technique.

Many meditation techniques practiced today come from ancient Eastern traditions. One of the more widely recognized forms of meditation in the West is Transcendental Meditation (TM), introduced to the United States by Maharishi Mahesh Yogi in the 1960s.

People who practice TM sit quietly, focusing on their breathing and repeating a single word or sound (sometimes called a *mantra*) over and over. The mantra is often selected for you by a meditation instructor, or guru. The traditional Sanskrit word used in meditation is "ohm," but you can choose any word or phrase you like. With practice, you learn to focus on the word or the sound itself and not on any conscious thoughts. If other thoughts do intrude, don't get distracted, frustrated, or upset. Simply acknowledge them and refocus on your chosen sound, word, or phrase.

Scientists at the Medical College of Georgia who've studied Transcendental Meditation have found that the technique decreases blood pressure by reducing constriction of the blood vessels, and thereby lowers the risk of heart disease.

Some people with fibromyalgia practice a very simple meditation technique to quiet the body and mind. It's so easy you can do it anywhere. Just breathe deeply and slowly and concentrate on a mental image of a tranquil object, such as a candle or flower. Simply gaze at the object for two minutes, then close your eyes while you continue to breathe deeply and see the image in your mind's eye. When you are ready to open your eyes, you'll feel refreshed and relaxed.

You can learn to meditate on your own by using self-help books, audiotapes, or videotapes, but a trained instructor can help you develop your skills more quickly. Each meditation session should last about 20 minutes, and you should aim for two sessions daily.

There are no national licensing requirements for instructors of meditation. Many hospitals, wellness centers, and continuing education programs offer classes and workshops.

GUIDED IMAGERY

Guided imagery, also called visualization, can help you control how you feel through the use of vivid mental pictures of relaxing situations, such as a beach, a waterfall, or a sunset. When used along with slow, deep breathing, guided imagery can reduce anxiety levels and lower your heart rate and blood pressure.

The technique has been shown to enhance the immune system in cancer patients, improve circulation in people with Raynaud's disease, speed postoperative recovery, and reduce stress in patients with irritable bowel syndrome, tension headaches, and so on. Some cancer patients, for example, feel empowered by using guided imagery during chemotherapy to imagine their white blood cells swallowing up tumor cells like Pac-man.

The technique is easy and you can do it anywhere. To get started, simply make yourself comfortable, close your eyes, take several slow, deep breaths, and imagine a tranquil setting. Take whatever time you need to construct an elaborate image of the place, full of physical and sensory detail. Now put yourself into the picture and experience the setting with all your senses. The more real your image, the more your body can convince itself that it's actually "there." What do you see? How does the air feel against your skin? What sounds and smells make the setting distinctive?

Next construct a visual metaphor that symbolizes the release of tension. If you're picturing a beach, for example, imagine yourself sitting at the water's edge, the waves coming into shore and rolling gently around your shoulders. As the waves recede, feel them pulling the tension out of your body and carrying it out to sea. Or imagine that you're a feather floating gently to the ground, the tension leaving your body as you drift downward. When you finally reach the ground, picture yourself as totally relaxed.

To relieve pain, first imagine that all your pain is contained in a ball of mercury. Now picture this liquid silver ball rolling down your arm or leg. Watch it roll across the floor and out of the room, leaving you pain-free. Or see yourself kicking it away as far as you can. You can also visualize the pain in physical terms, such as a burning fire. By mentally extinguishing the fire, you can sense an immediate lessening of pain.

You will notice that as you transport yourself to another place, your areas of pain and tightness begin to drift away. Continue to breathe deeply. When you're ready to return to the present moment, stretch your fingers and toes, even your entire body, and then open your eyes.

A professional therapist or commercial audiotapes can guide your visualizations and help open your mind to the power of subconscious healing. Guided imagery is often used in conjunction with other mind–body therapies such as hypnotherapy or biofeedback.

HYPNOTHERAPY

Hypnotherapy, or hypnosis, was recognized by the American Medical Association as a valid and effective medical therapy in 1957. Under hypnosis, you achieve a trance-like state in which you're susceptible to the power of suggestion. Some people use hypnosis as a way to cope with fears and phobias, manage stress, and ease pain. Hypnosis has been shown to be helpful for patients with fibromyalgia, irritable bowel syndrome, migraine headaches, or other painful disorders, warts or other skin conditions, asthma, and nausea.

Hypnosis can be used to control the pain and stress that go hand-in-hand with fibromyalgia. Patients who have tried hypnotherapy along with physical therapy have reported less pain, less fatigue, and better sleeping patterns than those patients who have received physical therapy alone.

If you're working on pain relief, the hypnotherapist will first have you concentrate on something other than your pain, and then will lead you through relaxation exercises. Once you are fully relaxed, the hypnotherapist might suggest images to help you experience your pain as something distinctly separate from yourself, a process known as dissociation. The hypnotherapist might also suggest that you think of the pain in a different way, perhaps as a warm or tingly feeling. This technique is known as *symptom substitution*. These methods can show you that it's possible to control pain and have a more positive, hopeful attitude.

There's no reason to be leery of hypnosis performed by an ethical practitioner. The technique is being used more and more in standard health care settings, especially to overcome negative habits such as smoking or overeating. When you're in a hypnotic state, you can have as little or as much control as you want at all times, and an ethical therapist won't try to make you do anything you wouldn't otherwise do. The technique simply helps you to banish negative thoughts and focus your mental energy on health and healing. If, for whatever reason, you can't find a hypnotherapist you're comfortable with, you can still experience the benefits of hypnosis using self-hypnosis techniques.

Most people can be hypnotized and some can even learn to hypnotize themselves, although it generally takes weeks or even months to learn to do it effectively. Many conventional physicians are trained in hypnotherapy, as are many dentists, psychotherapists, and nurses.

THE POWER OF PRAYER

Those who are scientifically oriented prefer to explain the healing effects of prayer through mind–body physiology, rather than entertain the possibility of a Higher Power. Whatever the mechanism at work in prayer, most health care providers no longer question its potential in helping people cope with chronic illness. Studies have shown that when patients with chronic disorders augment their medical treatment with some degree of "spiritual coping," they are less likely to become depressed.

In one study reported in the *American Journal of Psychiatry*, researchers studied 85 patients hospitalized with serious medical illness who had also become depressed. These patients completed a battery of tests, including the Hoge Intrinsic Religiousness Scale, which measures how deeply a person has internalized their religious values and faith. The higher the patient scored on this scale, the more quickly he or she recovered from their depression. This finding held even after accounting for improved physical health and any other factors that could have influenced recovery.

If your fibromyalgia symptoms have soured your outlook and mild depression is a constant mood state, consider the findings of a long-term study by the National Institute on Aging. This research established that people who attended one or more religious services each week were only half as likely to be depressed as those who attended less frequently or not at all. If you are comfortable with prayer, try to accept that there are some things we can never understand and put prayer to work for you on a daily basis, perhaps incorporating it into a program of relaxation exercises and/or guided imagery.

LOVE AND LAUGHTER AS MEDICINE

Did you ever hear the phrase "laughter is the best medicine?" Perhaps you've noticed that your pain seems to vanish when your mind and body are totally engaged in a good belly laugh.

Consider the case of Norman Cousins, the celebrated writer and editor who in the mid-1960s was diagnosed with an "incurable" form of arthritis known as ankylosing spondylitis, a severe condition marked by unremitting pain, stiff joints and spine, and a host of related disorders. Cousins was determined to fight the illness, not submit to it. He followed his doctors' orders for conventional treatment—mainly breathing exercises and medications—but he also tried an unorthodox therapy: humor. He watched slapstick movies, told jokes, and listened to jokes. And he discovered that the more he laughed, the better he felt.

In fact, Cousins maintained that his "laughter therapy" eventually cured him, and he described his experience in 1976 in the *New England Journal of Medicine*.

In the years that followed, scientists investigating this phenomena have concluded that just as stress and anxiety can raise blood pressure, upset the stomach, and tax the immune system and the heart, carefree laughter can calm the nerves, boost the immune system, enhance general body functioning, and—like soothing music—help a person cope with chronic pain.

Laughter can work wonders for the fibromyalgia patient, promoting healing by reducing stress, enhancing circulation, and lowering heart rate. There are important psychological benefits as well: Humor distracts you from unproductive, self-destructive thought patterns.

So rent some videotapes of classic TV and movie comedies, or listen to audiotapes of the great comedians. They may be just what the doctor ordered. Think of it as a part of your prescription for better health, and make laughter a priority every day.

Just as laughter heals, so does love. Bernie Siegel, a physician and professor of surgery at Yale University, has written several books focusing on the power of love to enhance wellness and help people deal with serious health disorders. I see it in my practice every day: The patient who can give and receive love freely is better equipped to ride out the ups and downs of chronic disease.

PET THERAPY

The companionship and unquestioning love and loyalty of a pet can be a real positive in the life of anyone with a serious illness. Even when you're aching and uncomfortable, it's hard to be completely miserable when you're greeted at the door by the sweet, upturned face of the family cat or the wagging tail and loopy grin of the family pooch.

Pet ownership can bring a number of health-enhancing benefits to people with fibromyalgia. Studies have shown that petting a dog or cat can actually lower stress levels. Not only that, the responsibility of walking a dog (a.k.a. "four-legged exercise machine") can get you up and out of the house and into the fresh air for some exercise. Just focusing on another's creature's needs for a while helps take you out of whatever you're feeling in the present moment, and that can be restorative in itself.

13

Putting It All Together: Stories from the Medical Front Lines

For every fibromyalgia patient, treatment should begin with a thorough history and a complete physical exam. In my practice, "thorough" means probing for problems in the six broad diagnosis/treatment categories I've described in this book. In other words, I look for signs of imbalance—structurally, biochemically, in movement, in the environment, in the mind–body arena, and energetically. Based on the findings of the history and the physical exam, I order appropriate lab tests.

Fortunately, most patients with fibromyalgia don't have imbalances in every category. In many cases a thorough evaluation reveals only one or two major areas that need to be addressed. In other patients there are multiple interrelated problems. The important thing is to understand that many different conditions can cause the same cluster of symptoms we call fibromyalgia.

Armed with this information I can begin to understand how each fibromyalgia patient is unique. It's this appreciation that allows doctors to craft individualized treatment plans. Taking a one-size-fits-all approach is a recipe for failure.

Just take a look at the following case reports.

MICHELLE

Michelle is a 22-year-old who, 18 months before I examined her, had come down with a flu-like illness accompanied by muscle aches and fatigue. Initially her doctor had treated her with antibiotics and this seemed to help for a time. Subsequent infections caused a flare-up of symptoms, but this time antibiotics did not provide any noticeable improvement. Her sleep was nonrestorative, she complained of foggy thinking, and she had some mild digestive complaints. Prior to her illness Michelle had been winning races as a competitive cyclist. Now she was barely dragging herself through daily activities. She had seen a number of specialists who did the usual assortment of tests, and all test results had been normal. The antidepressants, anti-inflammatories, muscle relaxers, and sleeping medication that had been prescribed were not bringing any relief.

When I examined Michelle I found she had multiple muscle tender points and her eyes were dull; otherwise she looked like the picture of health. All the tests I performed produced readings in the normal range, except for an elevated candida IgA antibody level consistent with overgrowth of candida in the mucus membranes of the bowel. I treated Michelle for this condition with dietary changes, supplements, and a prescription anti-fungal medication, but there was no improvement in her symptoms. Next I recommended traditional Chinese medicine (a combination of acupuncture and herbs), along with massage and a host of nutritional supplements, all to no avail.

Finally, we tried a series of intravenous Meyer's cocktail infusions once a week for four weeks. These infusions contain calcium, magnesium, vitamin C, and B vitamins. (Actually, the vitamin levels in the infusions were lower than what Michelle had been taking orally.) With these infusions, her urine changed color and so did her life. (Normally, heavy-dose B vitamins turn the urine to bright yellow or orange. With oral supplements there was no significant change in the color of Michelle's urine. However, after her first Meyer's cocktail, her urine showed the characteristic color changes.)

The weekend following her second Meyer's cocktail, Michelle's fatigue and muscle aches were significantly reduced. She placed third in a bicycle race. After the initial series of four infusions, we tried to maintain her gains through the use of digestive enzymes and oral hydrochloric acid to improve the absorption of nutrients. She did okay for a few weeks, then started to slide backwards. At this point, we did a series of six infusions which again produced dramatic improvements. For several months she did very well with only an occasional visit to the office for an intravenous booster, usually before a big race.

I subsequently lost touch with Michelle, but I can remember the brightness that returned to her eyes after the Meyer's cocktails allowed her to resume a zestful life.

What Can We Learn from Michelle's Case

Michelle's case illustrates two diagnostic "blind spots" common to conventional medicine—namely overlooking the possibility of candida overgrowth and not checking for subclinical malabsorption or wasting of nutrients.

Candida overgrowth is not unusual in patients with elevated sugar levels or in those who have been on antibiotics or steroids repeatedly. However, it's a controversial diagnosis that generates a great deal of hostility from skeptical physicians. Some doctors consider it an unproven and unverifiable pseudodiagnosis. At first, I was not a believer myself, because typically candida overgrowth is diagnosed on the basis of symptoms that are totally vague, subjective, and could be caused by any number of different conditions. However, since I felt that the only way to dissuade patients from believing in a pseudodiagnosis was to be armed with some objective data, I began ordering candida antibody tests. Much to my surprise, some of these patients actually *did* have very high candida antibody levels. Once they were treated with antifungal treatments, the levels came down and their symptoms improved.

In Michelle's case the treatment of yeast overgrowth, in and of itself, did not have any apparent clinical benefit.

Was it a red herring? Did the yeast overgrowth somehow impair digestion and absorption, and did the condition gradually improve after the imbalance was corrected and the digestive tract gradually healed? It would be easy to speculate, but I must admit I don't have definitive answers to these questions.

ALAN

Alan, a 44-year-old college instructor, endured muscle aches and pains for six years, which interfered with physical activity. Testing and treatment by an internist, neurologist, psychiatrist, and rheumatologist were unproductive.

When I saw Alan in my office his energy level was not too low, but he did complain of occasional poor sleep and trouble concentrating. I suggested several dietary changes as well as supplements to reduce muscle aches. After limited success with these approaches, we checked his DHEA-sulfate level and found it to be quite low. After starting a regimen of 25 mg of DHEA each morning, his DHEA-sulfate came up to the normal range and he was able to initiate and comfortably maintain a regular exercise program for the first time in years. Alan tried stopping the DHEA a couple of times, but each time his symptoms worsened. When he resumed the DHEA, his symptoms improved again.

Although Alan appreciated the improvement, he didn't feel he was totally restored to good health. A year later he spontaneously developed a superficial blood clot in a vein in his right leg. There had been no trauma to the leg or any history of obvious risk factors for clot formation. Since the condition was not dangerous, we simply treated the symptoms and the condition cleared. Shortly afterward he spontaneously developed another superficial clot, this time in a vein in his right forearm. At this point we did extensive tests for blood hypercoagulability. All of the tests were "normal," but I started him on Coumadin to dissolve the clots and prevent further clot formation. During the four months he was on Coumadin he felt great, back to his normal self. After stopping the Coumadin, some of his muscle aches returned, but not to the degree prior to DHEA supplementation.

In the meantime, in treating another patient with fibromyalgia, I had learned that some patients with fibromyalgia symptoms appear to clot too easily. I went back and reviewed Alan's blood tests and found that the PT (prothrombin time) and PTT (partial thromboplastin time) were both "lowish" (scraping the bottom of the normal range), and that the fibrinogen was "highish" (scratching the top of the normal range). These are exactly the types of changes you would expect in someone with subclinical hypercoagulability. Alan is now taking a tiny maintenance dose of Coumadin which keeps him at the high end of the normal range for PT, and once again he's feeling great.

What We Can Learn from Alan's Case

The two medical "blind spots" illustrated by Alan's case are adrenal exhaustion and subclinical hypercoagulability. The fact that Alan's symptoms abated with DHEA supplementation but returned when DHEA was stopped clearly indicated that low adrenal function was playing a role here. Generally, most doctors think in terms of "all or nothing" when talking about adrenal function. In other words, they recognize Addison's disease (the total nonfunctioning of the adrenal glands), and they recognize adrenal overactivity, but they do not consider underactive adrenal function to be clinically significant. With more and more research documenting the critical role of DHEA, the medical community should pay more attention to this important hormone and the glands that produce it.

Subclinical hypercoagulability (the kind that doesn't cause serious clots of the deep veins, the lungs, or in the arteries in the heart and brain), is for the most part not considered in the list of potential causes (a.k.a. "differential diagnosis" in medical circles) for fibromyalgia symptoms. The fact that we can see discernible patterns that suggest hypercoagulability even when all the blood clotting tests are "normal" shows that it can be a mistake to always rely on so-called normal ranges when looking for explanations. The normal range—one that encompasses 95 percent of the population—is determined by taking the mean in a given population, plus or minus two standard deviations. However, a reading that falls into the normal range for an entire population is not necessarily normal for any single individual. This is a very important distinction.

The lesson I learned in Alan's case was to pay close attention to even "normal" lab tests to see if there are abnormal patterns compatible with the patient's history.

"Normal" lab results can be a statistical delusion, one that encourages mental laziness. I also learned that subclinical hypercoagulability can contribute to fibromyalgia symptoms in some patients. Think of it as "angina of the muscles" due to reduced circulation in the tissues caused by an overactive clotting mechanism. Since my experience with Alan, I have identified several other fibromyalgia patients with this pattern, and most have responded well to low doses of Coumadin.

DEBBIE

Debbie is a 43-year-old woman who developed severe muscle aches and fatigue one year after her marriage 17 years ago. For a few years, she struggled to continue working as an accountant, but eventually her condition forced her to quit working outside of the home. Debbie also had difficulty doing domestic chores because they greatly exacerbated her symptoms. She had been treated by an allergist for allergies, an internist for hypothyroidism, a psychiatrist for her depression, and a rheumatologist for her fibromyalgia. None of these treatments had helped her pain and fatigue.

When I tested Debbie, I found that she had a low DHEA-sulfate level and elevated IgE and IgG food antibodies for dairy, wheat, and eggs. I started her on 10 mg of DHEA daily, and she modified her diet to avoid the highly reactive foods. With these measures in place, she had some mild improvement in her symptoms. At this point we added additional supplements, including calcium and magnesium, MSM (methysulfonyl methane), and grapeseed extract. She also began to use a biomagnetic mattress pad. These second-line interventions resulted in modest improvements in quality of sleep and reduced Debbie's pain, but the overwhelming fatigue was still present. At my suggestion she then tried acupuncture and massage, which provided some temporary relief.

Finally Debbie scheduled an appointment with a therapeutic touch practitioner in our office. After just one session, she experienced a dramatic increase in energy. Debbie is back hiking in the mountains and taking care of her family. Other than a couple of transient setbacks over the past couple of years, she continues to do well. Her case illustrates one model of recovery: small incremental changes in response to several interventions, and then a sudden, unexpected, and dramatic response—in this case, to therapeutic touch.

What We Can Learn from Debbie's Case

The role of food allergies in chronic illness is controversial, as is the testing methodology. Typically, allergists and immunologists are not fond of blood antibody tests for allergies. The relevance of elevated food antibody levels is disputed because avoiding these foods does not always result in clinical benefits. However, the same can be said of conventional skin allergy testing and desensitization.

Debbie seemed to have several biochemical/hormonal imbalances which, when corrected, led to modest improvements in her condition. However the most dramatic improvement came with the energetic technique of therapeutic touch. Therefore it seems that energetic imbalances can sometimes be more relevant and important than the usual biochemical markers that we rely on so heavily in Western medicine. Therapeutic touch is thought to correct subtle energy imbalances in the body. It continues to be a controversial therapy that critics and skeptics love to attack because they can't explain the mechanism of action. There is scientific research both supporting and discounting it. While we may not be able to explain how it works, the dramatic effects some fibromyalgia patients experience should make physicians sit up and take notice.

FRANK

At 35, Frank was exhausted. For the past five years the successful investment realtor had had to push himself through each day despite the gradual onset of fatigue, widespread muscle aches, difficulty concentrating, poor sleep, low body temperature, and decreased libido. For the last three years, he struggled to keep his high-performance career on track with regular visits to rheumatologists and neurologists. But conventional medical blood tests for anemia, autoimmune disease, infection, and thyroid function were repeatedly normal. And no medical treatments seemed to help.

In time, when Frank's fatigue and pain became so pervasive he could no longer perform at the level he thought necessary for his career, he sold his business and aggressively pursued alternative health approaches, including a better diet, stress reduction techniques, massage, and acupuncture. After two years of practicing these new lifestyle strategies, along with the use of various complementary therapies, Frank's condition had improved somewhat. But muscle pain and fatigue continued to limit his activities and keep him from resuming his high-energy life.

When Frank finally arrived in my office, he appeared quite healthy, with no obvious abnormalities upon physical examination other than the expected multiple muscle tender points. Testing revealed that he had a low free T3 level (the most active of the thyroid hormones and almost never tested for), a low DHEA-sulfate level (an adrenal hormone that is used as a building block for several other hormones, including testosterone), and a "lowish" testosterone level (toward the low end of what is considered the normal range).

I started Frank on a low dose of prescription Cytomel (T3), 5 micrograms (mcg) twice daily on an empty stomach, plus an over-the-counter DHEA, 25 mg daily in the morning. Blood work two months later showed a now normal free T3, and other thyroid functioning had stabilized. His DHEA-sulfate level had also improved but was still lowish, so we increased the dose of DHEA to 50 mg daily. After two months on this regimen, Frank's DHEA-sulfate and testosterone levels were both at midrange.

Just four months after being correctly diagnosed and properly treated for fibromyalgia, Frank regained his active life, without the muscle pains and fatigue that had limited him for years.

What We Can Learn from Frank's Case

Frank's history illustrates two "blind spots" of Western medicine—namely, the diagnosis and treatment of the thyroid and adrenal gland irregularities.

Patients whose blood tests reveal a normal TSH and T4 level but a low free T3 reading often suffer from Wilson's syndrome, a condition in which people make plenty of T4 but do not convert it very well to the much more biologically active T3. (This should not be confused with another, better known condition by the same name—a genetic disorder that leads to excessive accumulation of copper in the body.)

You can't diagnose Wilson's syndrome conclusively without checking a free T3 level. Since very few physicians ever order this test, it's no wonder the condition is often missed. Even among doctors who actively look for this condition, there are some who insist the blood tests are worthless and that the only accurate way to diagnose Wilson's syndrome is by checking axillary temperatures. According to this view, if your temperature readings are low, the diagnosis is confirmed. This view does not take into account that many other variables can cause a low body temperature, not just inadequate thyroid hormones. Physicians who adhere rigidly to the temperature protocol without checking blood levels invariably end up overtreating some patients, with potential for harm. Objective, verifiable lab data is key to good management of this syndrome.

Frank's low DHEA-sulfate level illustrates the adrenal exhaustion syndrome often seen in overachievers who are under chronic stress. Since the role of DHEA is more or less glossed over in medical school, very few physicians even think of testing for a DHEA level. Conjugated DHEA (DHEA-sulfate) levels are more stable and more useful as a screening test since they are not as subject to daily variations. If your doctor wants to check DHEA/cortisol ratios, then the DHEA-sulfate screening is not as useful.

Even though DHEA is available over the counter, it should be used only under medical supervision and only when the patient's history and lab tests indicate it is appropriate. Eventually, the FDA will probably take this and other hormones off the market, since there is no valid reason to allow the general public to have unrestricted access to hormones which can very easily be misused. Until then, the effects of DHEA supplementation should be monitored just like thyroid hormone or any other hormone. Patients who use it should be screened for hormone-sensitive tumors which could potentially be stimulated by DHEA.

Some practitioners advocate the use of adrenal, pituitary, and hypothalamic *glandular extracts* for this condition. The use of glandular extracts makes me very nervous for two reasons. First, glandular extracts available over the counter are totally nonstandardized and may vary wildly from dose to dose. The second reason is the growing concern over "mad cow disease" (BSE or bovine spongiform encephalopathy). I know of no glandular extract manufacturer that is taking specific precautions against transmission of BSE, other than claiming that the glands are harvested from free-ranging cattle.

SARAH

Sarah is a 52-year-old who four years ago was diagnosed with fibromyalgia, although her symptoms dated back approximately eight years. In Sarah's case, the body aches, nonrestorative sleep, and poor concentration had seemed to fluctuate with her menstrual cycle, worsening premenstrually. At the time that I saw her, she hadn't had a period in two years. She had unacceptable side effects (headaches, sore veins in the legs, and elevated blood pressure) from standard hormone replacement therapy (HRT), so she had stopped conventional HRT after a few months.

When I examined Sarah I found nothing remarkable other than multiple muscle tender points. Her blood work looked fine except for low female hormone levels, which came as no surprise since she was clearly menopausal. Because Sarah had a poor response to conventional HRT, I started her on a compounded natural estrogen product called Triest (composed of 80 percent estriol—the weakest of the three estrogens—10 percent estradiol, and 10 percent estrone), along with natural progesterone. She tolerated this form of HRT without problems. The quality of her sleep is much improved, she is mentally sharp, and her body aches are almost completely gone.

What We Can Learn from Sarah's Case

Sarah's case illustrates the role of hormone levels in perimenopause and menopause as contributing factors in some patients with fibromyalgia symptoms. For those patients who don't tolerate standard interventions, it's obviously better to have more therapeutic options, which allows individualization of hormone replacement therapy (or any therapy for that matter).

Even though Sarah met the textbook criteria for fibromyalgia, clearly an underlying hormone problem was causing her symptoms. This reinforces the notion that fibromyalgia is more of a descriptive term or label than a diagnosis in the truest sense of the word.

BILL

Bill is a 42-year-old who over the last eight months had developed extreme muscle pain, disrupted sleep, fatigue, and depression. He consulted a rheumatologist and neurologist who both agreed that he had fibromyalgia and that he had to learn to live with this condition. He began to take anti-inflammatories, antidepressants, muscle relaxers, and pain medications, but these were not particularly helpful.

When Bill came to my office I saw the obvious involuntary twitching of his muscles (called fasciculations), along with equally obvious muscle wasting. Upon questioning I discovered that he had lost nearly forty pounds since the onset of his symptoms. Blood testing revealed an elevated CPK (a muscle enzyme). A subsequent muscle biopsy and EMG/NCV (electrical nerve and muscle studies) were both abnormal.

The neuromuscular specialists here in Denver are now trying to figure out what Bill really has. It's clear the problem is serious, but it's also clear that it isn't fibromyalgia.

What We Can Learn from Bill's Case

Many different conditions can cause symptoms that mimic those of fibromyalgia. Even though fibromyalgia is a chronic condition, it's generally thought to be not particularly dangerous. However, there are times where the underlying problem can be very serious. Physicians need to be extremely thorough when evaluating fibromyalgia patients in order to avoid missing serious underlying disorders.

SHARON

Sharon is an obese 39-year-old office worker who gradually noticed more and more fatigue and general achiness over the years, to the point where the symptoms began to interfere with her work and her day-to-day activities. Her blood tests were normal, and the medications offered by the rheumatologist who diagnosed her fibromyalgia have only caused side effects without noticeable benefits.

When I took Sharon's history, she mentioned that she was sometimes awakened by her own snoring. We did a nocturnal pulse oximetry test (she simply wore a transdermal oxygen sensor on her index finger overnight) in her own home for minimal cost. This test showed she had sleep apnea (obstruction of the breathing passages while sleeping), causing impressive drops in her oxygen level while she slept. Sharon is currently using a CPAP machine (continuous positive airway pressure, which keeps the airways open) and she's feeling better. We are still working on reducing her weight.

What We Can Learn from Sharon's Case

Once again, we see that it's too easy to give some-one a label of fibromyalgia when important underlying conditions have not been diagnosed or addressed.

TAKING CHARGE AND MOVING AHEAD

In formulating a treatment plan for a chronic condition like fibromyalgia, it's generally best to start out with less aggressive interventions, those that you can actively control with diet, supplements, exercise, relaxation techniques, and by modifying your environment.

There are many advantages to being actively involved in your treatment. If you're passive, your physicians may have to resort to more aggressive thera-pies. More aggressive generally means more dangerous (because of a heightened risk of side effects) as well as more costly. If you decline the opportunity to take a more active role, it will be much more difficult to treat and correct the underlying conditions that contribute to your disorder. The goal we are seeking—to improve your quality of life—is much more attainable if you work with your health care team to make whatever changes are necessary in the environmental, dietary, and lifestyle areas.

BUILDING YOUR INTEGRATED HEALTH NETWORK

Self-help approaches are usually helpful but can only take you so far. There are times when additional therapies (CAM and/or Western medical interventions) are needed. Once again, the particular therapies you select will depend on your unique assessment.

Consider yourself fortunate if you can find all of the practitioners and physicians under one roof and working together in your best interest. In the absence of this type of collaborative team approach, you will need to take some initiative to identify credible practitioners (see Chapter 3) and establish and foster ongoing communications among your various health care providers.

The following list summarizes some of the complementary and alternative therapies that may be helpful:

COMPLEMENTARY/ALTERNATIVE THERAPIES

Energy Therapies such as therapeutic touch, healing touch, polarity therapy, reflexology, craniosacral therapy, Reiki, TCM (traditional Chinese medicine, particularly acupuncture and herbs), and homeopathy. Homeopathy is incompatible with most of the other energy therapies and thus should not be used simultaneously.

Structural/Musculoskeletal Therapies such as massage, chiropractic, and osteopathic. These can be quite helpful if performed gently by a practitioner experienced with fibromyalgia;

otherwise these approaches may actually aggravate symptoms and cause a setback.

Kinetic/Movement Therapies such as Alexander technique, yoga, and *tai chi*.

Nutritional/Metabolic Therapies such as dietary modification and the use of herbs and supplements. Nutritionists, herbologists, naturopaths, and Ayurvedic practitioners can all help provide individualized recommendations in this area.

Mind–Body Therapies including biofeedback, guided imagery, and stress reduction techniques.

WESTERN MEDICAL INTERVENTIONS

In general the Western medical therapies are more aggressive, more invasive, and have greater potential for side effects. However, there are several with a good risk to benefit ratio that may be helpful. See Chapter 2 for more information on these strategies.

Coumadin or *heparin*—if there is evidence of hypercoagulability

Florinef (fludrocortisone acetate)—in the morning or DDAVP (*desmopressin acetate*) in the evening, if the blood pressure tends to be low

Sinequan (doxepin)—at bedtime for sleep disturbance

Elavil (amitriptyline) or *Flexeril (cyclobenzaprine)*—at bedtime for sleep disturbance

Neurontin (gabapentin)—for chronic pain

Guaifenesin and *dextromethorphan*—for chronic pain

Lamisil (terbinafine) or *Diflucan (fluconazole)*—for systemic candida overgrowth

Nystatin—for mucosal candida overgrowth

Doxycycline, tetracycline, or *Biaxin (clarithromycin)*—for chronic mycoplasma infection

Natural hormones—to correct hormonal imbalances, if detected by testing

Thyroid medicine—with monitoring of blood tests to prevent overtreatment

DHEA and/or *pregnenolone*—with monitoring of blood tests to prevent overtreatment

Cortisol—titrated by blood testing to prevent overtreatment

Trigger point injections using lidocaine or *Marcaine*—for temporary pain relief

Intramuscular injections—B12, magnesium, B6, *Kutapressin* and others

Intravenous infusions of a Meyer's cocktail—which contains magnesium, calcium, vitamin C, and B vitamins

Growth hormone shots—if levels are low

FINDING YOUR WAY THROUGH THE MEDICAL MAZE

Given the broad array of options presented here, it's clearly to your advantage to find a physician with an integrative medicine perspective—someone who can guide you through the many choices, help you prioritize therapies, and monitor the effectiveness of each intervention. If the initial steps you take do not provide the relief you're looking for, then more aggressive interventions are always available.

100 WAYS TO FEEL BETTER RIGHT NOW

With a chronic disorder like fibromyalgia, you'll have good days and bad days. But even when things start to look a little bleak, it helps to remember that life is full of possibilities. Here are some simple ways to turn around a negative, self-defeating attitude.

- Do something you love to do.
- Write a thank-you note to someone who has made your life a little easier.
- Express your anger.
- Take a nap.
- Ask for help.
- Make a list of all the things you're thankful for.
- Keep a journal. Write down anything and everything that pops into your head.
- Buy yourself some flowers.
- Take a hot bath. Throw in some essential oils or herbs.
- Read a magazine.
- Go to lunch with someone special.
- Listen to your favorite music.
- Look at photo albums.
- Read a book with a child.

- Volunteer.
- Learn something new.
- Buy yourself or someone else something special.
- Call a friend or family member you haven't spoken with in a long time.
- Make time for that hobby of yours.
- Eat something wonderful or exotic for dinner.
- Put on your favorite outfit.
- Have a massage.
- Hug someone.
- Take a walk outside.
- Cry if you want to.
- Think of a realistic goal for the day and then work to meet it.
- Eat dessert before dinner.
- Find your sanctuary and visit it.
- Lie down in your yard and watch cloud formations.
- Look at the stars through a telescope.
- Listen to soothing music while doing gentle stretching exercises.
- Buy a new box of crayons and color in a coloring book.
- Better yet, draw *your own* pictures!
- Go to the park and feed the ducks or squirrels.
- Re-read a favorite classic.
- Go to a music concert or symphony.
- Forgive your parents.
- Clean out your clothes closet.
- Donate unwanted items to charity.
- Visit a museum.

- Go to a movie.
- Tell your children you love them.
- Sing.
- Read the comics.
- Get your hair cut.
- Volunteer your time in the maternity ward of a local hospital.
- Eat a Popsicle.
- Have a water balloon fight.
- Write a poem.
- Sit by a pond or lake.
- Go to the mall or airport and "people watch."
- Set up a tank and fill it with fish.
- Walk barefoot in the sand.
- Buy a hat.
- Plan a vacation.
- Dress up in your best clothes.
- Send a friend a card "just because."
- Watch old family movies.
- Do nothing!
- Go somewhere you've never been.
- Think about your three top physical attributes and feel blessed.
- Start and finish a puzzle—crossword, maze, hidden pictures, seek-a-word.
- Sit outside in the rain.
- Take your partner or child on a "date."
- Buy a new journal.
- Try a new food.
- Bake cookies.

- Eat those cookies.
- Draw on the sidewalk with chalk.
- Make a list of the top ten things that make you happy.
- Re-pot those plants.
- Hang a bird feeder in your backyard.
- Play a favorite board game with your family or friends.
- Make popcorn the old fashioned way—on the stove!
- Invent a recipe.
- Pull out high school yearbooks and wonder whatever happened to . . .
- Hire someone to clean your house, or at least to do the vacuuming.
- Visit a neighbor you don't know well.
- Listen to an audio book.
- Plant a window garden.
- Write a song.
- Teach your children a game of cards.
- Take an unplanned coffee or tea break.
- Play hookey from work for the day.
- Go to the park and watch children play.
- Say "I'm sorry" to someone who needs to hear it.
- Leave a tip for your newspaper carrier.
- Make a list of all the people in your life for whom you're thankful. Tell at least five of them.
- Wear two different-colored socks.
- Buy new bed sheets.
- Open all the drapes and curtains and lift all the shades in your home to let the sun shine in.

- Buy the soundtrack to your favorite movie.
- Tell your partner what you love most about him or her.
- Scream really loud.
- Take photos of your family.
- Share a secret about yourself with someone you trust.
- Help your child with homework.
- Meditate.
- Celebrate your un-birthday.
- Look in the mirror and smile; you have a lot to be thankful for!

ON THE HORIZON: THE FUTURE OF FIBROMYALGIA

Twenty years ago, the Fibromyalgia Study Club of the American College of Rheumatology had an average attendance of 10 at its annual meetings. In 1997, more than five hundred rheumatologists attended. In the early 1980s, less than $100,000 was being spent annually on fibromyalgia research. Today, we're spending $4.1 million, and we have every reason to believe the amount will increase.

In the next two decades, with more and better research, experts predict the body's pain pathways will be better understood, helping us answer such questions as:

- Why are some behavior patterns associated with pain amplification but not others?
- What does sleep have to do with growth hormone?

- Does muscle spasm result from a local reflex or does it come from signals within the spinal column?
- What really goes on inside a local tender point?

We may very well have customized exercise and conditioning programs for fibromyalgia sufferers that will be reimbursed by insurance companies. Information on how to improve self-esteem, decrease pain perception, and deal with depression related to fibromyalgia will likely be incorporated into the general training and education of mental health professionals.

With any luck, we'll have new classes of medicines to block Substance P and increase serotonin. Agents to stabilize the autonomic nervous system will be developed. And perhaps we'll even have vaccines against fibromyalgia-inducing infections.

The future definitely looks bright, and it's already starting to happen. Recently, doctors at the State University of New York's Health Science Center in Syracuse have begun to use positron emission tomography (PET) as a diagnostic tool to gauge the severity of a patient's pain. Similar studies are being conducted in other parts of the country and in Canada. Doctors are using imaging to observe brain cell changes resulting from stroke or spinal cord injury. And they are hoping for an explanation for the phenomenon known as "phantom pain," often experienced by people who have had a limb amputated.

Every step, large and small, brings us closer to the day researchers will crack the mystery of fibromyalgia and we can finally start treating not merely the symptoms but the underlying cause of this mysterious disorder. Even better will be the day when fibromyalgia is known only in history books.

Until then, we stand tall and do the best we can. Remember, *you are not your illness*. You are an explorer on an adventure, the captain of your own journey. Work with the best health care providers you can find, learn all you can, open yourself to new paths, and find your way. I know you can do it!

For More Information, Help, and Support

ON FIBROMYALGIA

American Fibromyalgia Syndrome Association
6380 E. Tanque Verde, Suite D
Tucson, AZ 85715
520-733-1570
www.afsafund.org

The Fibromyalgia Network
P.O. Box 31750
Tucson, AZ 85751
800-853-2929
www.fmnetnews.com
(This group publishes an excellent newsletter.)

WEB RESOURCES

FibroHugs—*www.fibrohugs.com*
Fighting with Fibromyalgia—*www.ps.superb.net/smessick/fms.htm*
Co-Cure Web Ring—*http://www.co-cure.org/cocurering.htm*
Comfort-U™ total support body pillow available through the Feel
    Good Catalog—*www.feelgoodcatalog.com*

ON RELATED CONDITIONS

American College of Rheumatology
1800 Century Place, Suite 250
Atlanta, GA 30345
404-633-3777
www.rheumatology.org

Arthritis Foundation
1330 West Peachtree Street
Atlanta, GA 30309
404-872-7100
www.arthritis.org

Arthritis National Research Foundation
200 Oceangate, Suite 440
Long Beach, CA 90802
800-588-CURE
www.curearthritis.org

Chronic Fatigue and Immune Dysfunction Syndrome
(CFIDS) Association of America
P.O. Box 220398
Charlotte, NC 28222-0398
800-442-3437
www.cfids.org

COMPLEMENTARY AND ALTERNATIVE CONTACTS

Acupuncture

Acupuncture.com
www.acupuncture.com

American Academy of
  Medical Acupuncture
5820 Wilshire Boulevard,
  Suite 500
Los Angeles, CA 90036
323-937-5514
www.medicalacupuncture.org

National Acupuncture and
  Oriental Medicine
  Alliance
14637 Starr Road, SE
Olalla, WA 98359
253-851-6896
www.acuall.org

National Certification
  Commission for
  Acupuncture
  and Oriental Medicine
11 Canal Center Plaza, Suite
  300
Alexandria, VA 22314
703-548-9004
www.nccaom.org

Acupressure

American Association of
  Oriental Medicine
433 Front Street
Chatasauqua, PA 18032
888-500-7999
www.aaom.org

Alexander Technique

American Society for the
  Alexander Technique
3010 Hennepin Ave South,
  Suite 10
Minneapolis, MN 55408
800-473-0620
www.alexandertech.com

Aromatherapy

American Alliance of
  Aromatherapy
P.O. Box 309
Depoe Bay, OR 97341
800-809-9850
www.205.180.229.2/aaoa

National Association for
  Holistic Aromatherapy
P.O. Box 17622
Boulder, CO 80308
888-ASK-NAHA
www.naha.org

Aston-Patterning

Aston Training Center
P.O. Box 3568
Indian Village, NV 89450
(702) 831-8228
*www.members.aol.com/
  SVUmassage/Aston.htmlf*

Ayurvedic Medicine

The Ayurvedic Institute
11311 Menaul NE, Suite A
Albuquerque, NM 87112
505-291-9698
www.ayurveda.com

Biofeedback

Association for Applied
Psychophysiology and
Biofeedback
10200 W. 44th Avenue,
Suite 304
Wheat Ridge, CO 80033-2840
800-477-8892
www.aapb.org

"Bogus" Therapies

Museum of Questionable
Medical Devices
www.mtn.org/quack/index.htm

National Council for Reliable
Health Information
www.ncrhi.org

Quackwatch
www.quackwatch.com

Bowen Therapy

International Head Office,
Australia
P.O. Box 733
Hamilton, Vic. 3300,
Australia
011-61-3-55723000
www.bowtech.com

Brain Gym
(Educational Kinesiology)

Educational Kinesiology
Foundation
1691 Spinnaker Drive,
Suite 105B
Ventura, CA 93001
800-356-2109
www.braingym.org

Chelation

American College for
Advancement in Medicine
23121 Verdugo Drive,
Suite 2704
Laguna Hills, CA 92653
714-583-7666
www.acam.org

Chiropractic

American Chiropractic
Association
1701 Clarendon Boulevard
Arlington, VA 22209
800-986-4636
www.amerchiro.org

International Chiropractors
Association
1110 North Glebe Road,
Suite 1000
Arlington, VA 22201
800-423-4690
www.chiropractic.org

Compounding Pharmacies

International Academy of
Compounding Pharmacies
P.O. Box 1365
Sugar Land, TX 77487
800-927-IACP
www.iacprx.org

CranioSacral Therapy

Upledger Institute
11211 Prosperity Farms Road,
D-325
Palm Beach Gardens, FL
33410-3449
800-233-5880
www.upledger@upledger.com

Feldenkrais
Feldenkrais Guild of North
America
3611 SW Hood Avenue,
Suite 100
Portland, OR 97201
800-775-2118
www.feldenkrais.com

Herbal Therapy
American Botanical Council
P.O. Box 144345
Austin, TX 78714-4345
512-926-4900
www.herbalgram.org

American Herbalists' Guild
P.O. Box 70
Roosevelt, UT 84066
435-722-8434
www.healthy.net/herbalists

Holistic Dentists
Holistic Dental Association
P.O. Box 5007
Durango, CO 81301
www.holisticdental.org

Holistic Medical Doctors
American Holistic Medical
Association
6728 Old McLean Village
Drive
McLean, VA 22101
703-556-9245
www.holisticmedicine.org

Holistic Nurses
American Holistic Nurses
Association
P.O. Box 2130
Flagstaff, AZ 86003-2130
800-278-AHNA
www.ahna.org

Homeopathy
The National Center for
Homeopathy
801 North Fairfax Street,
Suite 306
Alexandria, VA 22314
703-548-7790
www.homeopathic.org

Hypnotherapy
American Board of
Hypnotherapy
16842 Von Karman Avenue,
Suite #475
Irvine, CA 92714
714-261-6400
http://www.hypnosis.com/abh

Laboratories
Great Smokies Diagnostic
Laboratory
63 Zillicoa Street
Asheville, NC 28801
800-522-4762
www.gsdl.com

Meridian Valley Clinical
Laboratory
515 West Harrison Street,
Suite 9
Kent, WA 98032
253-859-8700
www.meridianvalleylab.com

MetaMetrix Clinical
Laboratory
5000 Peachtree Ind.
Boulevard
Norcross, GA 30071
800-221-4640
www.metametrix.com

Massage
American Massage Therapy
Association
820 Davis Street, Suite 100
Evanston, IL 60201-4444
847-864-0123
www.amtamassage.org

Associated Bodywork and
Massage Professionals
28677 Buffalo Park Road
Evergreen, CO 80439-7347
800-458-ABMP
www.abmp.com

Touch Research Institute
Department of Pediatrics,
University of Miami
School of Medicine
P.O. Box 016820 (Dept. 820)
1601 NW 12th Avenue
Miami, FL 33101
305-243-6781
www.miami.edu/touch-research

Meditation
Insight Meditation Society
1030 Pleasant Street
Barre, MA 01005
978-355-4378
www.dharma.org/ims.htm

Naturopathy
American Association of
Naturopathic Physicians
601 Valley Street, Suite 105
Seattle, WA 98109
206-298-0126
www.naturopathic.org

American Naturopathic
Medical Association
www.anma.com

Bastyr University
1307 North 45th Street,
Suite 200
Seattle, WA 98103
206-632-0354
www.bastyr.edu

National College of
Naturopathic Medicine
49 SW Porter
Portland, OR 97201
503-499-4343
www.ncnm.edu

Southwest College of Naturopathic and Health Sciences
2140 East Broadway Road
Tempe, AZ 85282
480-858-9100
www.scnm.edu

Nutrition
American College for
Advancement in Medicine
23121 Verdugo Drive,
Suite 204
Laguna Hills, CA 92653
949-583-7666
www.acam.org

The American Dietetic
Association
216 West Jackson Boulevard
Chicago, IL 60606-6995
312-899-0040
www.eatright.org

Osteopathy

American Academy of
Osteopathy
3500 DePauw Boulevard
Suite 1080
Indianapolis, IN 46268-1139
317-879-1881
www.aao.medguide.net

American Osteopathic
Association
142 East Ontario Street
Chicago, IL 60611
800-621-1773
www.aoa-net.org

Photoluminescence

Society for Light Treatment
and Biological Rhythms
842 Howard Avenue
New Haven, CT 06519
www.websciences.org/sltbr

Polarity Therapy

American Polarity Therapy
Association
P.O. Box 19858
Boulder, CO 80308
303-545-2080
www.polaritytherapy.org

Reflexology

International Institute of
Reflexology
5650 First Avenue North
P.O. Box 12642
St. Petersburg, FL 33733-
2642
727-343-4811
www.reflexology-usa.net

Reflexology Association of
America
4012 Rainbow Street,
K-PMB #585
Las Vegas, NV 89103-2059
www.reflexology-usa.org

Reiki

The International Center for
Reiki Training
21421 Hilltop Street,
Unit #28
Southfield, MI 48034
800-332-8112
www.reiki.org

The Reiki Pages
www.reiki.7gen.com

Rolfing

The Rolf Institute of
Structural Integration
205 Canyon Boulevard
Boulder, CO 80302
800-530-8875
www.rolf.org

**Therapeutic Touch/
Healing Touch**
   Nurse–Healers Professional
      Associates International
   1150 Roger Bacon Drive,
      Suite 8
   Reston, VA 20190
   703-234-4149
   www.therapeutic-touch.org

Thermography
   Aswhin Systems International
   P.O. Box 1014
   Dunedin, FL 34697
   727-785-5844
   www.home1.gte.net/infrared

Trager
   The Trager Institute
   21 Locust Avenue
   Mill Valley, CA 94941-2806
   415-388-2688
   www.trager.com

Yoga
   American Yoga Association
   P.O. Box 1986
   Sarasota, FL 34276
   941-927-4977
   *www.members.aol.com/
      amyogaassn*

OTHER RESOURCES

American Occupational Therapy Association
4720 Montgomery Lane
Bethesda, MD 20824
301-652-AOTA
www.aota.org

American Physical Therapy Association
1111 North Fairfax Street
Alexandria, VA 22314
703-684-2782
www.apta.org

COMPLEMENTARY/ALTERNATIVE MEDICINE WEB RESOURCES

Alternative Health News Online
www.altmedicine.com

Ask Dr. Weil
http://cgi.pathfinder.com/drweil

Colorado HealthNet
www.coloradohealthnet.org

Falk Library of Health Sciences, University of Pittsburgh
www.pitt.edu/~cbw/altm.html

National Center for Complementary and Alternative Medicine
www.nccam.nih.gov

New York Online Access to Health (NOAH)
www.noah.cuny.edu/alternative/alternative.html

INDEX

A

Aberrant muscle communication, 25–26
Acetaminophen, 136
Acquired immunodeficiency syndrome (AIDs) infection, 21
Acupressure, 231–33
Acupuncture, xiv–xv, 180, 228–31
Adenosine triphosphate (ATP), 137
Adrenal exhaustion, 76, 144–45, 312–14
Adrenal gland irregularities, 318
Adrenal tests, 76
Aerobic exercises, 170–71
Alcohol consumption, 180
Alexander technique, 44, 175, 290–91
Allergies, 153–55, 294
Allopathic medicine, 202
Alpha-linolenic acid, 116
Alternate healing systems, xiv
Ambien (zolpidem), 94
American Association of Naturopathic Physicians (AANP), 267–68
American Association of Oriental Medicine (AAOM), 230–31, 233
American College of Rheumatology, 72, 73
American Fibromyalgia Syndrome Association, 34, 186–88
American Naturopathic Medical Association (ANMA), 267
American Oriental Bodywork Therapy Association, 289, 290
Americans with Disabilities Act (ADA) (1990), 195
Angina, 294
Anthocyanins, 105
Antiarrhythmics, 97
Antiasthmatics, 97
Anticoagulants, 97
Antidepressants, 97
Antidiabetics, 97
Antihypertensives, 97
Antioxidant nutrients, 124–31
Anxiety, 13, 294
Arginine, 150–51
Arnica 30, 244
Aromatherapy, 253, 262–65
Arthritis, 141–44, 289

Aspirin, 254
Asthma, 294
Attitude, developing positive, 57
Autoimmune tests, 76–77
Ayurvedic approach, 103, 202, 224, 235–41

B

Back pain, 9, 11, 294
Balance, 226
Beta-carotene, 129
Biaxin (clarithromycin), 93, 326
Biochemical approaches, 44, 211, 253–68
Biofeedback, 294–96
Bioflavonoids, 105, 126–27
Biological rhythms, 145–46
Biomagnetic approach, 245–47
Biomagnetic mattress pad, 315
Biomagnetic therapy, 245–47
Biotin, 123–24
Blood antibody tests, 315
Blood hypercoagulability, 312
Blood testing, 321
Body, listening to your, 38–40
Bovine spongiform encephalopathy (BSE), 319
Bowen therapy, 279
Breathing, 172–73, 295
Bryonia 6, 244
B vitamins, 120–24

C

Caffeine, avoiding, 144–45
Calcium, 314
Calories, 109–10
Candida overgrowth syndrome, 77–78, 113, 157–59, 310–11
Capsaicin, 98–99, 140, 239
Carbohydrates, 111–14
Carotenoids, 105, 129–30
Carpal tunnel syndrome, 210
Cartilage extracts, 143
Celebrex (celecoxib), 95
Chakras, 236
Chamomile, 240, 255, 265
Chaparral, 257
Chi, 224, 227